Chronic Pain Evaluation

Chronic Pain Evaluation

A Valid, Standardized
Assessment Instrument

Karen S. Rucker, M.D.
Professor and Chair (Retired),
Department of Physical Medicine
and Rehabilitation, Virginia Commonwealth
University/Medical College of Virginia, Richmond

Foreword by
Paula Anne Franklin, Ph.D.
Research Project Officer (Retired), Division of
Disability Program Information and Studies,
Social Security Administration, Baltimore

BUTTERWORTH
HEINEMANN

Boston Oxford Auckland Johannesburg Melbourne New Delhi

Every effort has been made to ensure that the drug dosage schedules within this text are accurate and conform to standards accepted at time of publication. However, as treatment recommendations vary in the light of continuing research and clinical experience, the reader is advised to verify drug dosage schedules herein with information found on product information sheets. This is especially true in cases of new or infrequently used drugs.

∞ Recognizing the importance of preserving what has been written, Butterworth–Heinemann prints its books on acid-free paper whenever possible.

 Butterworth–Heinemann supports the efforts of American Forests and the Global ReLeaf program in its campaign for the betterment of trees, forests, and our environment.

Library of Congress Cataloging-in-Publication Data

Rucker, Karen S.
  Chronic pain evaluation : a valid, standardized assessment instrument / Karen S. Rucker ; foreword by Paula Anne Franklin.
    p. ; cm.
  Includes bibliographical references and index.
  ISBN 0-7506-7121-1 (alk. paper)
  1. Chronic pain—Measurement. 2. Chronic pain. I. Title.
  [DNLM: 1. Pain Measurement—methods—United States. 2. Chronic Disease—United States. 3. Disability Evaluation—United States. 4. Pain—United States. 5. Social Security—standards—United States. WL 704 R911c 2000]
  RB127 .R83 2000
  616'.0472—dc21

                                                                                          00-025645

British Library Cataloguing-in-Publication Data
A catalogue record for this book is available from the British Library.

The publisher offers special discounts on bulk orders of this book.
For information, please contact:

Manager of Special Sales
Butterworth–Heinemann
225 Wildwood Avenue
Woburn, MA 01801-2041
Tel: 781-904-2500
Fax: 781-904-2620

For information on all Butterworth–Heinemann publications available, contact our World Wide Web home page at: http://www.bh.com

10 9 8 7 6 5 4 3 2 1
Printed in the United States of America

Cover image courtesy of Social Security Administration Contract RFP #600-90-0229.

I dedicate this book to
my beloved husband David,
who has loved me and
carried me through sickness,
health, and this rigorous
project;

to Jesus Christ, my shield,
the lifter of my head,
through whom all things
are truly possible;

to my new son, Jason;

and to my patients with chronic pain,
who were the best teachers.

Karen Snowden Rucker, M.D.

The research behind this project was sponsored by the Social Security Administration under contract 600-90-0229. Additional research support was provided by the National Institutes of Health general clinical research centers at Virginia Commonwealth University/Medical College of Virginia (VCU/MCV) and the University of New Mexico (UNM). (VCU/MCV is funded by the Public Health Service under National Center for Rehabilitation Research (NCRR) grant MO1 RR 00065. UNM is funded by the Public Health Service under NCRR grant 5MO1 RR 00997-17.)

Contents

Appendices

Foreword

Americans have become accustomed to reaping the scientific benefits of major government projects. For the past three decades, the NASA program has been the outstanding example with its proliferation of commercial products that have enriched our daily lives. With the publication of this manual, the medical and scientific communities have the opportunity to use the comprehensive, multidimensional pain measurement instruments initially developed to improve administration of the Social Security Title II Disability Insurance and Title XVI Supplemental Security Income programs.

This manual documents how the Social Security Administration (SSA) Pain Assessment Instruments Development (PAID) project can meet clinical and research needs for an integrated, broad-gauged battery in diagnosis, treatment, and rehabilitation. Chronic pain continues to challenge all touched by it—patients, families, employers, insurance companies, health care providers, and government support programs. Musculoskeletal conditions increased in frequency from almost 13% of the 357,000 SSA disability worker awards in 1984 to more than 23% of the almost 588,000 disability worker awards in 1997. In the 14 years since the passage of the Social Security Disability Benefits Reform Act of 1984, the number of annual disability worker awards has increased 65%. The proportion of awards distributed because of pain increased 77%. Escalation is the most dominant feature in the pattern of chronic pain, as reflected in Social Security Title II disability program awards. For this reason, the word *timely* best describes the publication of this manual to assist health professionals in coping with this growth.

Science provides the keys to greater knowledge. Improved effectiveness and productivity come through systematic application of new knowledge. However, scientific research is a long-range, difficult, expensive, and comparatively rare endeavor. Therefore, it is gratifying to witness the extension of the benefits of the PAID project. It will reach a wider segment of the professional communities concerned with treatment and research related to restoring maximum functioning to persons with chronic pain and chronic pain syndrome. This manual signals the initial step in providing the tools requested by the 1987 Social Security Commission on the Evaluation of Pain and the 1988 National Academy of Sciences Institute of Medicine Committee on Pain, Disability, and Chronic Illness Behavior.

Paula Anne Franklin, Ph.D.

Preface

The Pain Assessment Instrument (PAI) is a multidimensional, multiperspective, comprehensive tool for evaluating chronic pain. It has been tested on more than 1200 people with chronic pain and found to be a valid, reliable, and accurate predictor of likelihood of return to work. The first version of the PAI included every question possible that may have been predictive of return to work by persons with chronic pain. Most items deemed as not reliable or invalid were eliminated. Although some items were not particularly reliable or valid, they were retained because the clinical and research teams believed these items were important in a comprehensive database on chronic pain.

The Social Security Administration described the scientific work performed on this project in the following excerpts from Dr. Paula Franklin, project officer, in her project evaluation [emphasis added]:

> The performance of the PAID contract needs to be assessed in relation to the challenge of the work that
>
> - required *creative intellectual "cutting edge" interdisciplinary, academic work* by highly trained professionals to develop pain assessment tools for administrative instead of clinical use;
> - was a contract with tight agency control setting rapidly paced deliverables. These focused the complex research sequence over an extended period. Customarily this type of research endeavor is funded by a grant allowing the investigative team autonomy and the leisure of proceeding at their own pace and direction; and
> - had few precedents upon which to build. *Many leaders in the field said pain measurement for SSA disability determination was impossible to accomplish.*
>
> The contract award was based on the quality of the technical proposal from the research team. ... The design was scrutinized, passing the judgment of professional peers at a series of scientific conferences during the contract period. The PAID work has gained acceptance and recognition in the scientific and medical communities.
>
> The body of pain research completed during the 44 months not only *created new pain measurement tools, it broke new conceptual ground for pain and functional assessment.* ...

The PAID research administration and coordination has been remarkable given the complexity of each study. Most difficult has been locating and following the samples of persons with chronic pain, particularly in the national study with SSA disability applicants. Locating and following this population with limited information and less accessibility has been a feat in itself. ...

I rate the performance first class, the products of the highest quality.

This manual provides information on how the PAI was developed through Social Security Administration research contract RFP 600-90-0229. Information is provided on how to use the forms, complete the forms, and handle potential problems or questions that may arise.

The PAI as provided in this manual does not allow the user to predict return to work because the software necessary to do that without a large mainframe computer has not been developed. We plan to develop this software because it makes the PAI even more useful and adds a new dimension to the assessment of, management of, and decisions made about persons with chronic pain.

At a minimum, use of the PAI will provide a comprehensive valid reliable database on chronic pain patients. The future utility and potential of this unique tool is exciting.

Comments and suggestions for improvement are welcomed. Please contact:

Karen S. Rucker, M.D.
Principle Investigator, PAID Research Project
Director, Pain Assessment Instrument Project
P.O. Box 13584
Richmond, VA 23225
E-mail: ksrucker@mindspring.com

Acknowledgments

It is important to acknowledge many of the professionals who conducted medical chart reviews in cramped clinic quarters; made thousands of telephone calls to screen potential research volunteers; tracked medical records; monitored and synchronized the schedules of patients, physicians, and evaluation facilities; arranged transportation when needed; performed the evaluations; conducted the interviews; searched for research subjects 6 months after the clinic visit and chronic pain disability determination; searched computer rolls for missing subjects; and ultimately managed and entered the data on more than 1400 participants. A data pool of more than 2500 Social Security Administration (SSA) claimants was created for the national validity phase that was stratified to mirror as closely as possible the SSA disability recipient population. Still others wrote the computer programs that allowed closely monitored data management, designed the data screens for simplicity of data entry, and performed the statistical analyses.

Virginia—Virginia Commonwealth University Sports Medicine Center, Pain Management Center, and the NIH General Clinical Research Center, Department of Physical Medicine and Rehabilitation, Research and Training Center on Supported Employment:

Shirley Anderson	Karen Drilling
Trisha Baker	Tim Elliott
Dave Banks	Tom Florian
Kevin Billings	Katie Funk
Pam Brown	Howard Garner
Phil Bryant	Sharon Gilley
Ralph Buschbacher	Christy Gilman
Lois Buschbacher	Bill Hedrick
Mary Carruth	Ana Hernandez
Kern Carlton	Chris Hinnant
Chuck Chermside	Thomas Hock
Andi Conti-Wyneken	Donna Kinder
Kathy Dec	Sandy Kramer
Rick DeCarlo	Greg Leghart

Tom Lum   Maureen Skahan
Burnell Maddox   Rhonda Smith
Susan Marhon   Stefanie Tran
Billie Martin   Darlene Unger
Pat McGowan   Lou Usry
Bill McKinley   Debby Valenti
Barbara McNeil   Bill Walker
Karen Newman   Chris Walker
Betty Prince   Mary Wells
Amir Rafii   Ming Zhu
Faye Richardson   Wil Zuelzer
Chuck Silvers

A special thanks to Marie (Helen) Metzler. As research coordinator for the project, she was invaluable. She provided creativity, kept us in line scientifically, and was a real trooper during the long days and nights of this project. Steve Conley, project coordinator, also worked hard to keep us all organized and to make the project fun. Invaluable technical guidance was provided throughout the project by Paul Wehman and John Kregel.

Support from the leadership of VCU/MCV was critical to the timely completion of this work. I thank Steven Ayers, Dean; Eugene Trani, President; John Cardea, Chairman of the Department of Orthopedics; and Dick Keenan, Chairman of the Department of Anesthesiology, for their unwavering support.

Pennsylvania—Thomas Jefferson University Hospital and the Crozier/Chester Hospital

Peggy Abrams   Donna Loughran
Robert Condin   Gerda Maissell
John Ditunno   Patrick Murphy
John Graver   Edie Rosalie

Missouri—Jewish Hospital at Washington University Medical Center

Jeffrey Anderson   Richard Roettger
Paul Bates   Tracy Spitznagle
John Mikuzis   Oksana Volshteyn

Illinois—Illinois Transition Project of Southern Illinois University

Jim Bronkema   Craig Miner
Terri Clough   Jim Murphy
Hank Graver

New Mexico—University of New Mexico General Clinical Research Center and Albuquerque Veterans Medial Center

Kathy Dieruf
Katie Funk
Stanley Geel
Linda Kopriva
Asja Kornfeld

Charles Kunkel
Susan LeFebre
Kathy Legosa
Jorge Tapia

Indiana—Indiana Center for Rehabilitation Medicine and Indiana University at Purdue University in Indianapolis

Lynnette Green-Mack
Diane Hollinden
John McGrew
Mark Reecer

Michelle Salyers
Bob Silbert
Kathy Strong

Washington—Virginia Mason Medical Center and the Harborview Regional Epilepsy Unit of the University of Washington

Tom Curtis
Robert Fraser
Dave Koepnick

Trish Murphy
Mary Kay O'Neil
Faren Williams

DDS Regional Offices
Joni Albright, Indiana
Frank Jost, Sharon Houchins, and Cecily Barker, Missouri
Richard Fairbanks, New Mexico
Howard Thorkelson, Pennsylvania
Russell Owens and Jack Carraher, Virginia
Ed Davis and Don Barger, Washington

Social Security Administration and the Disability Determination System:

Gerry Abbott
Richard Bell
Charles Bishop
Peggy Burcker

Susan David
Wayne Harrison
Alan Shafer
Joe Tanzi

Finally, I thank Paula Franklin, our outstanding project officer. It is impossible to fully account for the depth and degree of support and assistance this remarkable person provided to our efforts.

Although I am sure to have overlooked some of those who helped lead this complex effort to its successful end, I have attempted to recognize those who provided assistance over almost 4 years of intensive and vital work.

Consultants to PAID Research Project

Gerald Aronoff, M.D., Director, Boston Pain Center

Sung Choi, Ph.D., VCU/MCV Professor of Biostatistics

Karen Drilling, R.P.T., Supervisor, Outpatient Physical Therapy, MCVH

Tim Elliott, Ph.D., VCU/MCV Psychology

Albert Farrell, Ph.D., VCU/MCV Professor of Psychology

David Florence, M.D., Vice-president of Medical Affairs, Polyclinics of Harrisburg, Pennsylvania; member of the original Pain Commission, recommended to PAID by the chair of that commission

Stephen Harkins, Ph.D., VCU/MCV Anesthesiology and Geriatrics; researcher in the areas of pain assessment and geriatrics

Harold Merskey, D.M., F.R.C.P., Director of Research, London Psychiatric Hospital, London, Ontario, Canada; founding member, International Association for the Study of Pain. Before the National Predictive Validity phase, we worked with Dr. Merskey to analyze the components of the overall instruments as we entered the final phase of data collection.

Otto D. Payton, Ph.D., VCU/MCV Professor of Physical Therapy

Donald Price, Ph.D., VCU/MCV Anesthesiology; member of editorial board of *Pain,* the journal of the American Pain Society

Amir Rafli, M.D., Director, VCU/MCV Pain Management Center

Joel Silverman, M.D., Professor and Chair, VCU/MCV Psychiatry

Max A. Woodbury, Ph.D., M.P.H., Emeritus Professor of Biomathematics for the Center for Demographic Studies at Duke University

(All affiliations are listed as they were at the time of the study.)

Social Security Administration Advisory Panel

Lowell Arye, Income Security Policy Office of the Assistant Secretary for Planning and Evaluation

Thomas Drury, Ph.D., Deputy Director, Epidemiology and Oral Disease Prevention Programs, National Institute of Dental Research

Terrence Dunlop, Ph.D., Office of Medical Evaluation

Rosemary Hall, Division of Field Disability Operations

Gerald Hendershot, Ph.D., Chief of Illness and Disease Branch

Stephen Jencks, Office of Research, Health Care Financing Administration

Armand Lefemine, M.D., Director, Surgical Service 112, Department of Veterans Affairs

Virginia Miller, M.D., Technical Assistance Office, Office of Workers Compensation Programs

Guy Moody, Division of Medical and Vocational Policy

Lynne Penberthy, M.D., M.P.H., Office of Research, Health Care Financing Administration

Raymond Seltser, M.D., Center for General Health Services Extramural Research Agency for Health Care Policy and Research

Eleanor Walker, Health Science Administrator, Center for General Health Service Extramural Research, Agency for Health Care Policy and Research

(All titles are listed as they were at the time of the study.)

Chronic Pain
Evaluation

1 | Development of the Pain Assessment Instrument

COMMISSION ON THE EVALUATION OF PAIN

In March 1987 the Commission on the Evaluation of Pain published a report for the U.S. Congress and the Department of Health and Human Services. This assembly of professionals from multiple disciplines identified the most important areas of social science investigation in pain, pain assessment, and disability. The Commission on the Evaluation of Pain found a general lack of knowledge and understanding of chronic pain and pain behavior and lack of a comprehensive database on chronic pain and Social Security Administration (SSA) disability claimants. It found that SSA tools and techniques for obtaining information about pain are inadequate. One of the primary recommendations was for the SSA to develop scientifically the tools to remedy these findings.

The commission recommended the early stages of disability determination be redesigned to obtain better information about pain and pain behavior by redesigning forms to alert interviewers and adjudicators to cases in which pain is a substantial element and by developing questionnaires to collect more information about pain at the earliest opportunity in adjudication. They found that because legal statutes and regulations are standard across the nation, assessments and data collection also should be standard.

In 1988, the SSA awarded a contract to develop a pain study design and to draft test instruments for subjective measurement of pain, categorization of pain claimants, and prediction of return-to-work potential. Drafted questionnaires were delivered in December 1988 and formed the starting points for this research contract.

In 1989, the SSA released a request for proposal to conduct the research study to revise, test, and formally develop these tools scientifically through assessment of a large number of persons with chronic pain. This research contract, for the Pain Assessment Instruments Development (PAID) project, was awarded to Virginia Commonwealth University in June 1990, with Karen S. Rucker, M.D., as the Principal Investigator, and was completed in 1994.

FEDERAL REGULATION REVISIONS

After the contract was awarded in June 1990, additional and revised SSA pain regulations were proposed. These new regulations were published for comment, reviewed, and amended by the SSA in November 1991.

The 1991 regulations followed the general trend to define disability in terms of functional abilities and major life activities. The move to functional considerations in these assessments fostered additional impetus for standardized measurement methods and assessments to help determine the effect of pain on a person's ability to work.

Another major development during the 44-month period the studies were underway was the passage of the Americans with Disabilities Act of 1990 (ADA). This major civil rights initiative for persons with disabilities expands the Civil Rights Act of 1964 and the Rehabilitation Act of 1973. It is steeped in individual employment considerations and defines disability in terms of major life activities. In the ADA, *disability* is defined under the standard that the disability determination must include physical or mental impairments that substantially limit one or more major life activities of an individual. Under the ADA, major life activities include but are not limited to "caring for oneself, performing manual tasks, walking, seeing, hearing, learning, and working." This functionally based definition specifically identifies these primary activities of daily living as the standard for the determination of who qualifies under the ADA as having a disability.

The move to a more functional interpretation of impairment is driven by the national debate on our health care system and resources. Outcome measures are becoming more common in the assessment of the efficacy of medical and rehabilitation interventions. Functional improvement may soon become the defining reimbursement level for some procedures. Data showing long-term results of treatment could become the basis for specific criteria for alliance organizations to develop contracts within the new health plan reforms.

PAIN ASSESSMENT INSTRUMENT DEVELOPMENT PROJECT

It is generally acknowledged that pain is a multidimensional phenomenon. No single comprehensive pain measurement instrument has spanned the breadth of data available from the instruments described and presented in this manual. The successful development of the Pain Assessment Instrument (PAI) through the SSA research contract RFP #600-90-0229, known as the Pain Assessment Instrument Development (PAID) project, has made an important contribution to a massive health policy problem. There are now reliable and valid multidimensional assessment instruments for chronic pain that accurately predict likelihood of return to work. Testing of the instrument has been repeated in a multicenter national study involving the SSA claimant population, and the instrument has been revised on the basis of the results of the analysis.

The instrument described in this manual is called the *Pain Assessment Instrument (PAI)*. It was previously called the *Multidimensional Multiperspective Pain Assessment Protocol (MMPAP)*. The MMPAP was the original scientific product from the national multisite final validity study. The name MMPAP was also used in two published scientific papers (see Chapters 6 and 7).

Changes to the PAI, in the future, if any, will be made so as not to change the validity. Studies will have to be conducted to ensure maintenance of validity, and users will be notified as to the effect of these changes on the validity of the instrument.

The most important aspect of changes to the PAI that affect validity is in the prediction of likelihood of return to work. Use of an equation on the data collected by means of the PAI and comparing it with data from a national sampling of SSA disability claimants with pain has been found to predict likelihood of return to work with 87% accuracy. In the smaller, earlier validity study involving approximately 600 general pain patients 18 to 65 years of age, the likelihood of return to work was predicted accurately 90% of the time (the population was adjusted to compensate for the overabundance of low back pain).

PURPOSE OF THE PAIN ASSESSMENT INSTRUMENT

The Pain Assessment Instrument (PAI) was developed to provide a valid, reliable, multidimensional, and standardized pain assessment battery that can be routinely and uniformly used to facilitate the assessment of pain in disability determination. The instruments that compose the PAI have been piloted and scientifically validated through a nationwide study. Construct validity has confirmed distinct domains related to pain. Concurrent validity analyses, in which use of the component area was comparatively measured with use of previously validated instruments, have confirmed that the instruments measure the areas they are intended to measure.

Use of these instruments should allow standardized data collection for the disability application process that includes specific and predictive questions on chronic pain. This is important because some persons with trauma or other disabling conditions do not report pain at their initial application without being asked specifically whether pain is present. Likewise, during disability determination, applicants may develop subsequent or secondary chronic pain conditions. If pain is considered in a standardized manner, each separate application or reconsideration will identify pain as a factor at the beginning and at each subsequent phase of application. Pain has not been identified or examined separately by the SSA in the past, as emphasized in the SSA definition of disability: "inability to engage in any substantial gainful activity by reason of *any medically determinable physical or mental impairment* which can be expected to result in death or which has lasted or can be expected to last for a continuous period of not less than 12 months" [italics in original].

In addition to use in disability determination, it is anticipated the PAI will be a valuable clinical tool that will aid in both the objective and subjective assessment of chronic pain. The forms developed for this protocol standardize assessment of this critical area by medical staff. They provide a comprehensive, routine measure not previously available and replace the anecdotal or case-by-case interpretations typically used. The physician form provides a framework for the physician to obtain specific information, which guides physicians to make informed, objective recommendations.

At this point in time, the PAI provides a structured and carefully developed format for collecting comprehensive data on patients with chronic pain. Physicians who use the PAI will have a guideline for ensuring that all information has been collected on every patient. A key focus of the data collected on the instruments is likelihood of return to work; therefore the focus is on the *functional impact of chronic pain on the person.*

The information collected includes the following:

- Amount of pain
- Functional performance estimates
- Potential for rehabilitation
- Impact of pain on ADLs
- Laboratory and other diagnostic support or lack thereof for current diagnosis
- Issues related to return to work

This information can be entered into a computer program to provide a database or onto paper records. It can be used to answer questions from insurance representatives, case managers, lawyers, and other involved parties.

The PAI can be completed both before and at the conclusion of treatment to determine variables that indicate effectiveness of treatment. The PAI, however, is not intended to be used to provide the "end all" answer. Physicians should use the PAI as they would other diagnostic tests and clinical assessments to contribute to their assessment and recommendations for a given patient.

IMPLICATIONS

A major need identified by the Commission on Evaluation of Pain, the Institute of Medicine, and the SSA has been for a valid, reliable multidimensional assessment tool for persons with chronic pain. The great need for a rational and consistent decision-making process concerning chronic pain and disability is apparent. Inconsistencies exist in physical examinations, history-taking techniques, and interpretation of examination and history findings for chronic pain. In this time of limited resources and increasing expectations, decisions must be made regarding resources for persons with chronic pain (disability benefits, access to pain treatment centers, rehabilitation, and so on), and they are being made on a daily basis. Physicians are being asked to provide information and recommendations by workers compensation carriers, federal agencies, and the judiciary system. These groups have varying levels of training, knowledge, and experience about pain and disability. In the past, there was not a consistent or rational data collection to support or guide the decisions. These decisions ultimately affect psychosocial, physical, and economic aspects of patients' lives and the economics of business, industry, and government.

The implications of the development of this standardized protocol are far ranging. The PAI has potential as a comprehensive data collection tool and as a measure of treatment effectiveness. Use of the PAI will allow comparison of outcomes at various pain treatment centers. The PAI has been proved to be a valid and reliable pain assessment protocol that encompasses all domains related to chronic pain assessment within one multiperspective tool. Additional research is needed to confirm and extend the results of current investigation. Research possibilities include demonstrating the therapeutic and diagnostic utility of the protocol. It is expected that use of the PAI will improve responsiveness and decision making among the various parties who manage and assess chronic pain.

The purpose of this manual is to make the PAI available to the scientists, clinicians, and private disability insurance companies and to describe the background, development, and testing. Clinically useful information for implementation of the PAI in an office or administrative setting also is included.

Future editions of this manual and the PAI will provide computer software and the equation used in the national study, use of which allowed a prediction success rate of 90.2% (see Chapter 3). The equation for predicting return to work must be transferred from a mainframe computer to more user-friendly software.

I hope that presentation of the PAI in its current form makes it useful for the general pain population on a national level. With feedback from the users of this manual, future editions will be aimed at providing a more user-friendly format.

Uses for the Pain Assessment Instrument

DEFINING CHRONIC PAIN

The inability to meet adult role expectations because of chronic pain represents a large and growing problem. Functional limitations due to pain disrupt the lives of thousands of individuals each year and challenge the nation's health care system and work force when left to operate efficiently despite loss of human resources. In a recent poll of Americans concerning their experience with severe pain, nearly one fourth of adults said that they experienced pain strong enough to interfere with their daily activities every month.[1] Eighty-three percent of respondents in another study reported persistent pain that had lasted longer than a year.[2] For employed persons with pain, the result has been more than $55 billion a year in lost work days.[3]

Chronic Pain and Chronic Pain Syndrome

Chronic pain is defined as *pain persisting beyond the expected healing time of an injury or an illness, usually considered beyond six months.* Chronic pain is also frequently referred to as chronic intractable pain or chronic nonmalignant pain, according to the American Medical Association *Guidelines for Evaluation of Permanent Impairment.*[4]

Chronic pain improperly diagnosed or inadequately treated can result in deteriorating coping skills. Under such circumstances, persistent chronic pain results in progressive limitations and reductions in functional capacity. These problems can contribute to the evolution of the chronic pain syndrome. Thus, chronic pain represents the nidus of chronic pain syndrome.

Chronic pain syndrome is a complex condition with physical, mental, emotional, and social components (Figure 2-1). Both chronic pain and chronic pain syndrome can be defined in terms of duration and persistence of the sensation of pain. Psychological and emotional components may or may not be present. However, chronic pain syndrome, as opposed to chronic pain, has the *added* component of certain recognizable psychological and socioeconomic influences (Table 2-1).

Although there may be some blurring of the boundaries between chronic pain and chronic pain syndrome, the characteristic psycholog-

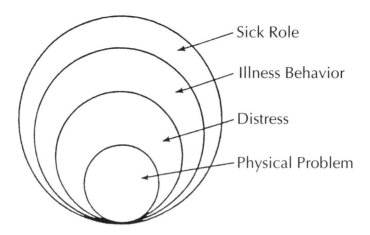

Figure 2-1 The Glasgow Illness Model. The biopsychosocial concept of illness. (Reprinted with permission from Waddell G, et al. Chronic low-back pain, psychological distress, and illness behavior. *Spine*. 1984;9:209–213.)

Table 2-1   Difference between Chronic Pain and Chronic Pain Syndrome

Sign or Symptom	Chronic Pain Syndrome	Chronic Pain
Pain lasting more than 6 months	Yes	Yes
Objective physical findings	Yes/No	Yes/No
Pain behaviors	Yes	No
Overuse of health care	Yes	No
Substance abuse	Yes	No
Magnification of symptoms	Yes	No

ical and sociological behavior patterns inherent in chronic pain syndrome distinguish the two conditions. Within the framework of this definition, chronic pain may exist in the absence of chronic pain syndrome, but chronic pain syndrome *always* presumes the presence of chronic pain.

Pain behaviors are the hallmark of chronic pain syndrome and include the following:

1. Willingness to undergo repeated diagnostic studies, which generally are inconclusive and contradictory
2. Willingness to undergo repeated therapeutic procedures, which usually result in temporary reduction in pain and often only make the patient worse
3. Overutilization of the health care system, evidenced by a high frequency of physician visits as the patient becomes dependent on the physician

4. Frequent changes in health care professionals, described as "doctor shopping"
5. Body language displays such as grimacing and bracing

Pain behaviors frequently make the patient seem difficult for the physician to treat, and because "everything else has failed," the physician refers the patient for either a surgical procedure or for a psychiatric visit, thinking the problem must be "in the patient's head." Pain behaviors are evidence of a syndrome and should cue the physician to refer the patient to a comprehensive and multidisciplinary pain management program that might have been appropriate as an earlier treatment strategy.

Pain behaviors have many reinforcers. For some, continuation of pain (and pain behaviors) is rewarded with attention and increased concern from significant others. Pain may provide a legitimate rationale for leaving an undesirable work environment. For some, medical attention provides authenticity and "rewards." These instances provide subconscious feedback in which suffering and pain behaviors occur in large part because "good things" happen as a result of the behavior.

Pain behaviors can be very dysfunctional and limiting. They contribute to changes in interpersonal relationships and activities of daily living. Left untreated, they result in dependency, loss of social and family roles, depression, and other psychological problems. Substance abuse, in the form of abuse of prescription drugs and alcohol, is a frequent stigma of patients with chronic pain. Persons with chronic pain syndrome lose the ability to function properly in many areas of their lives because of their chronic pain behavior and the associated loss of coping mechanisms, rather than solely because of the underlying pathologic condition. It is important to understand, however, that although the emotional and psychological features described are components of chronic pain syndrome, these individuals *do not have psychogenic, unreal, or imaginary pain.* Chronic pain syndrome *must be differentiated from malingering and other serious emotional disorders.* The Commission on the Evaluation of Pain has stated that chronic pain syndrome is not a psychiatric disorder.[5]

An important differentiation for chronic pain is that persons with chronic pain but without chronic pain syndrome may also lack objective physical findings and may claim disability due primarily to pain. However, these persons, without the associated pain behavior, continue to function well in emotional and social spheres despite the pain. They may exhibit poor endurance but are functional. For example, they can sit and stand but perhaps not for periods sufficiently long to be productive. They can walk; however, pain may cause them to stop after a short distance. They may be limited in the distance they can carry heavy loads or in the duration of performing a task.

Such individuals have usually worked for many years despite their pain, but physical alterations and changes in posture, gait, or work-related motions or efforts have become more obvious. This pain may eventually limit their productivity and longevity in the workforce. However, they do not exhibit pain behaviors, thus differentiating them from patients with chronic pain syndrome. For both chronic pain and chronic pain syndrome, the greatest socioeconomic impact of the person's alteration in function is on the ability to work.[2,5,6]

Malingering is defined as the conscious and deliberate feigning of an illness or disability. *Malingering involves the fabrication of symptoms and complaints in order to achieve a specific goal.* There is consensus among pain specialists and the Commission on the Evaluation of Pain that malingering is readily detected with appropriate medical and psychological tests. The Social Security Administration (SSA) estimates that frank malingering is present in less than 1% of SSA disability claimants. The PAID study revealed the same results. Approximately 1% of patients were felt by study physicians to be malingering.

Magnification or exaggeration of symptoms must be differentiated from malingering. Patients with chronic pain may magnify or exaggerate symptoms for many reasons aside from the simple feigning of an illness or disability. Patients may magnify their symptoms to gain recognition of their pain, which otherwise may not provide objective findings. Patients may feel a need to magnify their symptoms in order to be believed and to receive the attention they feel is appropriate for their suffering.

A physician's recognition of magnification of symptoms *should not invalidate* the patient's complaint. Instead, magnification of symptoms should give the physician additional information regarding the patient's perception of his or her problems and psychological state. In fact, magnification of symptoms may represent pain behaviors in many patients and must be treated along with the physical findings. It is important to differentiate physical findings from pain behaviors in order to more appropriately and comprehensively direct treatment. An example is shown in Table 2-2.

Pain behaviors are not necessarily untreatable and should not be viewed as a permanent condition. Rehabilitation for chronic pain syndrome may include behavioral modification training.

Table 2-2   Example of Difference Between Physical Findings and Pain Behaviors

Physical Finding	*Pain Behaviors*
Loss of passive ROM	Guarding
	Creating loss of active ROM and resistance to passive ROM although full motion can be obtained with relaxation or positioning

ROM, range of motion.

The Commission on the Evaluation of Pain[5] has recognized pain as a "complex experience with social and psychological factors complicating attempts at measurement" and developed a set of criteria to assist in categorizing persons who exhibit chronic illness (pain) behavior. Although the statutory authority of the Pain Commission, given by Congress, has since expired and has not been reauthorized, these criteria provide a method of identifying persons who exhibit chronic pain behavior. One of the primary components of the PAID study was to assess the validity of these criteria for the assessment of disability with a consideration of pain.

To meet the selection criteria the individual must meet criteria for *pain* and *effects of pain,* as follows:

A. *Pain,* as evidenced by:
   1. *Measurable impairment of function with physical tissue damage in body parts specifically related to the complaints of pain.* This is specifically assessed in the medical examination portion of the physician and patient pain assessment instruments.
   OR
   2. a. *Pain complaints apparently disproportionate and/or inappropriate in location, intensity, or duration to the physical damage and/or its normally expected healing time.* The specification of "disproportionate" requires interpretation by physicians only, because they are the only persons who have the experience to assess the proportionality of the applicant's complaints.
   AND
      b. *Behavioral manifestations of pain, which must include THREE (3) of the following:*
         (1) *Preoccupation with pain as evidenced by persistent and repeated complaints or willingness to undergo repeated painful diagnostic or therapeutic procedures in search of a cure.* This is a combination of the factual historical representation by the claimant ("What medical procedures have you had performed?") as well as a subjective assessment by the physicians.
         (2) *Overutilization of the health care system as evidenced by frequency of physician visits or surgical procedures or frequent changes of health care professionals.* This is also a combination of the factual historical representation by the claimant and the subjective assessment by the physicians.
         (3) *Persistent excessive use of analgesic and/or sedative drugs.* All parties involved are questioned about medications. An assessment also is attempted of recreational drugs and drug dependency.

(4) *Consistent audible and body language displays such as grimacing, bracing, guarding movements, or disturbances of station or gait as observed by physicians, interviewers, associates, family, and other observers.* All parties involved are asked to assess body language and movement displays.

(5) *Other accepted, objectifiable pain-related behaviors such as sleep disturbances, eating disorders, or sexual dysfunction.* This category is by its very nature global and spans all forms.

B. *Frequent and/or persistent episodes of ALL of the following due to pain:*

1. *Marked restriction of activities of daily living.* This includes activities such as cleaning, shopping, cooking, and other general activities of daily living. The physician and patient are asked to give an assessment.
AND

2. *Marked difficulties in maintaining social functioning.* This refers to the capacity to interact appropriately and communicate effectively with others. This includes the ability to get along with others and is assessed by all involved.
AND

3. *Failure to complete tasks in a timely manner.* This refers to work-related functions such as concentration and persistence. Again, all parties involved assess the applicant's abilities.
AND

4. *Marked restriction in objectifiable functional capacity to perform basic work activities.* The patient and both physicians estimate the applicant's functional abilities.

THE NEED FOR PAIN ASSESSMENT

When the Pain Assessment Instrument (PAI) was being designed in 1989, payments from the disabled workers' entitlement program (Social Security Disability Insurance) totaled $11.2 billion. By 1992 the total had increased to $17.7 billion or more than 58%.

The backlog of pending claims at the end of 1989 was 479,000. In 1992, the backlog was 725,000 with an average waiting period of 12 weeks for claims to be processed.[7] This is the number of weeks of work pending in the Disability Determination Service (DDS) offices and produces the best approximation of the amount of time an applicant must wait for an eligibility decision. Assessment of the impact of chronic pain on disability is critical for a variety of reasons and historically has increased the time spent on adjudicating claims; many of which go on to the administrative law judge (ALJ).

The many goals associated with assessment and measurement of chronic pain are reflected in the variety of directions pain assessment research and the development of pain assessment tools have taken in recent years. The primary goal of most chronic pain assessment, as with acute pain, is as a diagnostic tool.[4,8,9] To obtain relevant diagnostic information on individual patients, clinicians use short questionnaires, checklists, or other devices, many of which they have developed themselves[10,11] or which they have modified or compiled on the basis of existing instruments.[12] From these instruments comes the goal of determining treatment effectiveness, often measured by changes in pain or reported pain levels. Brief but easily repeatable assessment tools such as the visual analogue scale (VAS),[13] the Functional Independence Measure (FIM),[14] and the Oswestry score,[15] have been used to document the effectiveness of various treatment protocols. Last, a valid and reliable accurate pain assessment tool will meet the goals of assessing function[16] and predicting functional abilities[17] and related consequential actions, including disability assessment,[18,19] workers compensation, formalized pain research,[20,21] and pain treatment center evaluation.[22]

Ambiguities in assessment strategies and variation in examinations used to identify physical or mental impairments have led to increased litigation related to disability involving pain.[23,24] Variable judicial rulings have led to congressional concern that a standard for assessing pain in disability determination should be established judicially rather than administratively and be based on sound scientific and medical information. This concern precipitated Section 3 of Public Law 98-460,[25] which put into statute the longstanding pain policy of the SSA and called for the appointment of a Commission on the Evaluation of Pain[5] to work in consultation with the National Academy of Sciences Institute of Medicine[2] to evaluate the policy for evaluation of pain and recommend appropriate changes.

Chronic pain and its definition are problematic because of a lack of consensus about basic definitions and inconsistencies in measurement and assessment techniques. Although considerable effort has been put into a taxonomy to help classify various pain symptoms,[26,27] at present no classification system for chronic pain, musculoskeletal disorders, or back pain (the most common subgroup of chronic pain) is uniformly used. Because pain is subjective and not directly measurable, prior assessment efforts have focused on a wide range of standard diagnoses and etiologic indicators, patient self-reports, physician rating scales, and psychological assessment tools. With few exceptions,[28–30] most diagnostic tools and forms for chronic pain assess a single domain. Many instruments are used as a subjective assessment of pain frequency, length, intensity, and unpleasantness; psychological perception of pain; pain behaviors; perception of control over pain; and pain interference with sleep.[31–33] Other instruments specifically assess mental health status, such as the patient's self-report of depressive symptoms, contact with the mental health system, substance abuse, and sociopathy.[34–36] Some instruments address the patient's social support network, including support provided by the patient's significant other and the significant other's reaction to the patient.[37] Diagnostic protocols used to record medical information related to the physical examination may also include health care utilization, use of medication, diagnosis, and cause of pain.[38,39] Functional limitations are measured as the effect of pain on the patient's concentration and cognitive processes, activities of daily living, emotional status, and functional abilities as perceived by the patient and physicians.[14,40,41] Employment history and vocational rehabilitation potential are assessed less frequently but are deemed important with respect to treatment outcomes.[42,43]

The wide array of areas investigated during pain assessment has necessitated use of a variety of approaches. Both the patient's perspective and the physician's perspective seem crucial in assessment of the multiple dimensions of the patient's pain. Subjective measures, such as patient self-report and physician interpretation, are essential additions to the objective information obtained by the physician through a physical examination. However, all instruments currently in use reflect a single approach, such as the patient's subjective perspective,[44,45] the physician's subjective perspective,[15] or objective physical measurements.[39,40]

The forms developed for the PAI standardize assessment of all these critical areas by medical staff and persons with chronic pain and provide a routine measure that prevents case-by-case interpretations. The physician form provides a framework for the physician to obtain specific information that allows the physician to make an informed, objective recommendation regarding the pain claimant.

WHO SHOULD USE THE PAIN ASSESSMENT INSTRUMENT?

It is anticipated that the PAI will be a valuable clinical tool that will aid in the both the objective and subjective assessment of chronic pain. The PAI provides a level of standardization that would be desirable for SSA and for other government programs. Use of the PAI, if mandated for existing administrative systems, could streamline implementation. Many SSA disability recipients are processed through the workers compensation arena before they apply for SSA benefits. Therefore, the instruments could be added to a state's workers compensation and long-term disability programs in an effort to standardize disability and pain assessments; something not currently available in most states. Utilization of a standardized pain assessment instrument would make it possible for claimants and agencies to document pain and the functional impact of pain before they reach the SSA.

Because the number of pain treatment centers is increasing throughout the nation, a consistent assessment of chronic pain is a growing need. Present assessment strategies and subsequent outcomes among treatment centers are not directly comparable. The varied methods used at pain treatment centers to assess pain preclude comparison across centers.[41,46,47] Other facilities that must evaluate factors related to chronic pain are struggling with the same problem of lack of comparability. The use of a standardized protocol would alleviate this problem. A vital need has therefore been identified for a valid and reliable multiperspective, multidimensional pain assessment tool.[48]

Chronic Pain Treatment Centers
Chronic pain has always been challenging to physicians and health care providers from the standpoint of definition, classification, diagnosis, and treatment. Whether the health care professional is a physician in solo practice or a psychologist who is part of a structured treatment team, comprehensive, consistent data collection is required. The need for physicians to determine the presence of permanent impairment and to give recommendations regarding likelihood of performing functional tasks and returning to work has multiplied the challenges presented by persons with chronic pain. For physicians to address these needs, a great deal of information must be obtained and factored into medical decision making. Such information can be gleaned from a variety of areas, including the following:

- Psychological status
- Coping mechanisms
- Social supports
- Vocational issues
- Functional performance
- Motivation
- Rehabilitation potential
- Mental health
- Behavior

Many of these areas are unfamiliar territory for most physicians because traditional medical school and postgraduate training programs do not provide education about chronic pain or these associated medical areas. As was suggested by literature and experience with physicians across the nation in the multisite final validity phase of the PAID project, physicians have different ways of evaluating chronic pain. Inconsistencies exist in physical examinations performed, history-taking techniques, and interpretation of the findings for chronic pain. Given this, it is not surprising that there is wide variation in impairment ratings and disability assessments.[15,39,40,44,45] Even among professionals who are educated and trained in chronic pain, there remains wide variation in interpretation of physical examination findings, the implications of the data obtained for the treatment plan, and the gathering of psychosocial and vocational information.

The availability of a comprehensive, valid, and reliable assessment tool for chronic pain is critical in capturing the multidimensional information required for these patients. Standardization of assessment provides treatment centers with the potential to compare patient populations and outcomes internally, regionally, and nationally. The comprehensiveness of the PAI and the inclusion of the elements most likely to predict return to work along with the multidimensional elements are critical and unique features.

Additional affirmation of the need for a standardized instrument and the ability of this instrument to fill this need was demonstrated when a number of the physicians who participated in the PAID study asked to implement the forms in their personal clinical practices. These medical professionals believed that the instruments assured them of addressing all necessary areas for patients with chronic pain.

Workers Compensation System

It is apparent that there is a great need for rational and consistent decision making in chronic pain and disability. Physicians are being asked by workers compensation carriers, federal agencies, and the judiciary system to provide information and recommendations. These groups have varying levels of training, knowledge, and experience about pain and disability. Workers compensation rules vary by state. Even in the federal program of SSA disability determination there has been no consistent data collection to support or guide decisions.

Returning injured workers to work, identifying appropriate and effective treatment interventions that will help return the worker to the job, and accurately predicting whether a worker will be able to work in the future are issues asked of physicians on a daily basis. The answers are critical for the workers compensation carrier and the injured worker. Once compensation and disability decisions are made, there is no longitudinal tracking system in place to assess the impact of these decisions. These decisions ultimately affect psychosocial, physical, and economic aspects of patient's lives, and they impact the economics of business, industry, and government. The PAI can be used to track longitudinally the functional, clinical, and administrative outcomes of these populations.

Social Security Administration Disability Determination Service

The Report of the Commission on the Evaluation of Pain[5] emphasized the need for a standardized evaluation of chronic pain, in particular, for disability-related decisions:

Since disability requirements for eligibility are set down in the law, all claimants must be evaluated under the same criteria. At the same time, the disability program consists of several levels of adjudication and a large body of trained disability examiners and medical and legal professionals responsible for the decision making. To maintain a national program, a *standard* for the evaluation of pain that can easily be accepted, understood, and applied by the large body of adjudicators at all levels of adjudication is essential.

Additional reasons given by the Pain Commission for standardized instruments in the data gathering on and assessment of pain in the consideration of disability included the following:

1. Given different claimants with similar medical-vocational profiles, like decisions should be made.
2. The same rules should be applied regardless of where a person resides.
3. Different adjudicators, given the same set of facts, should reach a similar conclusion.

Because we are dealing with legal statutes and regulations that are standard across the nation, the assessments and data collection also should be standard and consistent. Use of the PAI provides standardized forms for the comprehensive assessment of chronic pain. In the current version, the forms are designed to be field tested in the disability application process. Implementation of the PAI in SSA depends on results of such a study of SSA disability procedures as a whole.

Because the standardized instruments have predictive utility, use of these forms should help avoid the variations in interpretation of disability criteria now experienced with each separate case as it goes before an ALJ in the advanced stages of an appeals process. At present applicants have to wait until the final stage of appeals for the ALJ to interpret pain behaviors. With the PAI these behaviors can be recorded and the applicant's personal experience presented with measured observations of this subjective area by trained physicians. The forms offer a standardized assessment of this critical area by medical staff and provide a consistent method of measurement that prevents case-by-case interpretation by an ALJ.

FUTURE USES

The PAI, as presented in this manual, provides the ability to collect comprehensive, multidimensional, multiperspective data on persons with chronic pain in a standardized manner with a scientifically proven valid and reliable instrument. The clinical and research potential for the utility of the PAI is significant and includes the following possibilities:

1. Predicting likelihood of return to work
   - as compared with the SSA disability applicant chronic pain population
   - as compared with the national chronic pain population
   a. Clinical outcome measurement tool
   b. Research tool for measuring treatment effectiveness
2. Establishment of a national database on persons with chronic pain
3. Utilization in SSA disability determination

1. Predicting Likelihood of Return to Work
Factors involved in determining whether a person with chronic pain will return to work are varied and complex. Some persons who exhibit chronic pain behaviors without objective physical findings are able to function adequately in an employment situation for an extended period of time. Other persons who exhibit the same pain behaviors may over time lose their ability to cope with the physical, social, and psychological demands of work and permanently remove themselves from the workforce. The specific factors that predict or contribute to whether an individual will be able to remain productive in the face of chronic pain and/or return to work after an extended absence due to pain has been a matter of intense investigation.

The published body of research on chronic pain and predicting return to work overwhelmingly emphasizes unalterable variables such as demographics and work history. Understanding that the SSA would not wish to emphasize these characteristics in the determination of disability, the PAID project conducted a discriminate function analysis without these variables. Therefore, the predictors that have emerged from this study are more directly related to the areas that chronic pain may affect, such as an individual's physical limitations, basic functional abilities, and psychological or behavioral factors.

To predict return to work outside the scientific setting, software must be developed for data entry and for use of the equation currently on the main frame computer at Virginia Commonwealth University. Once the software has been developed, tested, and distributed, the utility of the PAI will have significant clinical and research implications.

Utilization of the PAI allows clinicians to accurately and consistently assess data elements that affect the likelihood that persons with chronic pain will return to work. Early medical evaluation of these data elements (physical limitations, basic functional ability, and psychological or behavioral factors) could impact treatment plan choices. For example, patients identified as not likely to return to work could receive psychological intervention, vocational assessment, comprehensive rehabilitation, or behavioral intervention sooner than they would otherwise receive them. Ideally, use of appropriate clinical interventions earlier would improve clinical outcomes and timing of return to work. Identification of unaddressed problem areas for workers compensation patients is key to returning patients to work. Although the software for predicting return to work from the data collected with the PAI is not available for dissemination at present, this instrument would still be a very valuable tool for workers compensation insurers. Requiring the PAI to be completed for specific populations of workers compensation injuries could produce considerable cost savings in the long term and improve care for injured workers. Such populations could include all back and spine injuries and any musculoskeletal injury for which the patient is not back at work within a specified time. For example, a worker with an injured shoulder remains out of work for 4 weeks. The carrier requires that the PAI be completed by a trained physician. This gives the carrier direct data regarding physical examination findings and social, psychological, and vocational issues that may be affecting this worker's recovery.

Use of a proven battery such as the PAI could also assist with reimbursement issues. Every physician has had patients who needed a more comprehensive approach or specific interventions earlier in the course of treatment to increase the likelihood of returning to work. The battle of convincing third-party payers of the need for such interventions often is a difficult and unsuccessful one. Use of and education about a proven assessment tool may go far to support physicians' recommendations for intervention and improve return-to-work rates.

In 1993, Martin[49] blamed the "high tech, high cost health care system" for unnecessary interventions by doctors and their attraction to expensive technology. The PAI involves no expensive or high-tech equipment. It is simply a structured, multidimensional questionnaire.

The PAI could be used to assess the effectiveness of rehabilitation interventions. Patients identified by means of a valid and reliable instrument as not likely to return to work could be assisted in finding interventions that would change the outcome predicted. Use of these instruments in medical rehabilitation research to assist in proving what works would be very valuable, particularly at a time when third-party payers are demanding proof that expensive interventions are effective. Prediction of likelihood of return to work will require software and application of the equation used in the research study. The instrument provided in this manual allows one to collect comprehensive and function-oriented data that are valid and reliable.

2. National Database
The current database created for the PAID study contains data on more than 1300 persons with chronic pain. Most of the individuals were followed up with 6-month interviews and when possible with 12-month interviews. This database contains extensive demographic and

pain-related information and will provide a fruitful research source for multiple post hoc research questions. It must be pointed out, however, that the database required stratification constraints that preclude generalizations about persons with chronic pain in general. Therefore, it is not intended to be epidemiologic in nature.

With dissemination of the PAI and development of user-friendly software, a large national database could be developed for bench marking. This would offer many options for data evaluation and access.

3. Use in SSA Disability Determination

The SSA disability determination offices could use the PAI to determine disability for those not likely to return to work. This would eliminate time-consuming and expensive appeals and readjudications. The existing process has often resulted in eventual awarding of benefits through the courts. However, these benefits usually are awarded several years after the initial application, only after an ALJ had the benefit of seeing that the claimant has not returned to work in the interim. In these cases, the process delays distribution of benefits to pain patients and creates additional costs for the SSA.

Perhaps another use of the PAI by the SSA would be to identify claimants who need early vocational, psychological, or behavioral interventions. To assure effective utilization, the PAI would require field testing in the SSA disability determination environment.

USER-FRIENDLINESS OF THE PAIN ASSESSMENT INSTRUMENT

Important to the success of the PAI is its user-friendliness. Ease of administration and interpretation of data will impact its use and the completeness and accuracy of the data. The user-friendliness of the current PAI format can be improved. The current format was developed to meet scientific criteria necessary for conducting reliability and validity testing. For the next edition of this manual, I hope to receive feedback nationally from PAI users as to what changes would meet their needs. In addition, work will be progressing on developing clear data-entry fields for software and changing the PAI visual format to be more clinically useful in the physician's office.

The key to making any changes to the forms is to be assured of retaining the reliability and validity. Additional testing must be conducted with any substantial changes made. The same issue exists for using shorter versions of the PAI. Although we can identify items that are most predictive of return to work and we can narrow these to the bare minimum required, we will not know the effect of the physician who does not collect data in the areas eliminated from the instruments. We believe that through the process of collecting data on the *complete* PAI, the physician obtains the information that allows accurate completion of the key elements that predict return to work. This, however, will be an issue later, when the software is available for use in predicting return to work.

At this time, the PAI is a valid and reliable, comprehensive data collection instrument that ensures the gathering of vital information on chronic pain. It can be used to establish a database on populations of patients with chronic pain and allow comparison of data between diagnoses and treatment outcomes. This will provide data for health insurance companies, workers compensation agencies, disability determination agencies, and providers of short- and long-term disability benefits.

CHAPTER

3 | Scientific Validation of the Pain Assessment Instrument

OVERVIEW OF THE SCIENCE BEHIND THE PAIN ASSESSMENT INSTRUMENTS

Because pain is subjective and not visible to others, the science behind the Pain Assessment Instrument (PAI) is critical. There are no universally accepted ways to measure and assess pain. The key is how pain affects one's life, including ability to work, interact with others, and fulfill the expectations of society. The U.S. government and private agencies have policies to assist those who cannot provide for themselves due to illness or injury. The difficult question is how to distribute limited benefits to those in need. Persons with chronic pain have long been at the end of the list, neglected because of the subjective nature of the illness.

When it comes to providing financial resources, science is accepted when a person's word is not. In the area of chronic pain, many assessments are available to determine the various characteristics behind the pain, and their impact, but few have sound, defensible science behind them. Defensible science is essential in these days of litigation and bureaucracies.

The statistical information presented herein is detailed, as is often the nature of statistics. Some portions were written specifically to provide scientific defense to expert statisticians. From the moment of conceptualization of this project—the development of comprehensive instruments to assess chronic pain to predict return to work—the need to have sound scientific procedure was starkly recognized. The entire project was conducted in anticipation of defending the science in court and proving to critical scientists and statisticians that these instruments can be used accurately and consistently to predict whether a person returns to work. With this in mind, the results obtained with the PAI were scrutinized carefully by scientists, Social Security Administration representatives, and peer reviewers of scientific journals. Experts from all over the United States specializing in areas of pain, statistics, psychology, mathematics, and various other medical specialties acted as consultants on all aspects of the development and testing of the PAI.

The purpose of the detailed statistical discussion is to provide a resource to those who use the PAI and may need to defend their use of it to make clinical decisions and recommendations from its data. A glossary of statistical terms is provided. Key statistical points are as follows:

1. **Data and information were collected in the following specific domains:**
   - *Rating of pain dimensions*—how pain is described and perceived, whether pain interferes with sleep
   - *Medical information*—how the patient uses or overuses health care services, whether the patient is willing to tolerate medical procedures for managing pain, physical examination findings, effectiveness of pain treatments, results of medical testing, medications used
   - *Mental health*—the patient's emotional status, presence of depression or substance abuse
   - *Social support networks*—the availability of family and friends who provide help, understanding, and emotional support
   - *Functional limitations*—how pain affects the ability of the patient to perform activities, to function
   - *Employment and rehabilitation*—willingness of the patient to work, willingness to make accommodations and changes to be able to work, need for rehabilitation

2. **The questions on the PAI are accurate in the collection of information in these areas.** The PAI has been compared with other proved and accepted instruments for collection of information in similar areas and has been proved accurate in collection of similar information (*concurrent validity*).

3. **The information collected with the PAI is consistent and accurate** (a) when collected by the *same person* from the same patient repeatedly over time (*test-retest reliability*) and (b) when collected by *different persons* from the same patient (*interrater reliability*).

4. **The PAI, when used with computer software and an equation, is accurate for predicting the likelihood someone will return to work.** Predictions were calculated with a computerized equation from data collected with the PAI. The patients were contacted 6 months after completion of the forms. Which patients returned to work and which did not had been accurately and consistently predicted with the equation and the PAI data (*predictive validity*).

EXPERT PANEL

A number of expert consultants participated in development of the PAI and in modification of the instruments after each research phase.

The consultations were obtained to ensure that the design included the most necessary elements of evaluation. Consultants participated in two formal roundtable discussions and studied various functional and statistical reviews as the studies progressed. In the summer of 1990, the first roundtable included investigators in pain assessment from Virginia Commonwealth University (VCU) and several other prestigious institutions. The first effort significantly modified and expanded the baseline instruments.

When the pilot study was completed, another roundtable was held in January of 1992. The purpose of the second roundtable was to reduce the size of the instruments before the reliability and validity testing phase of the study. This session led to the final instrument design used in the main portion of the study. This meeting reduced the total instruments 25% from the original, pilot test versions.

Throughout the analyses conducted at the end of each phase, internal statistical consultants were enlisted to ensure appropriate statistical techniques and interpretations. The project was aided by an internal SSA Advisory Panel composed of leaders of SSA and related federal representatives whose agencies and divisions were affected by the need for valid and reliable pain assessment instruments. We were fortunate to have available the experience of these government employees who served on the internal advisory panel.

INITIAL PILOT STUDY

The PAI started with instruments drafted by Chronic Illness Care Inc. through a 6-month SSA contract. Researchers at VCU conducted an extensive literature review and added items identified in the two roundtable reviews. This initial development and expansion ensured that the PAI expanded on earlier research and addressed shortcomings identified. The goal was to begin with a comprehensive instrument that included every potentially predictive variable. During this phase, the number of items on the instruments increased 200%.

Data were collected from a variety of perspectives. Patients supplied basic demographic and vocational information on an initial referral form and completed a subjective assessment instrument that contained information about pain experienced at the time of completion of the form and in the past. Two physicians performed a physical examination and completed a form containing both subjective and objective information, including treatment history. The comprehensive list of forced-choice items was initially pilot tested with 67 patients who had reported pain for at least 6 months. Components that could not be consistently and repeatedly assessed were dropped from the battery.

The research study was designed in three distinct developmental phases: (1) **pilot**, (2) **reliability and early validity**, and (3) **national**

final validity. Each phase directed both the structure of the next phase and the composition of the research test instruments in the subsequent phases. Each phase is discussed with a description of its purpose, design, sample, and results.

Sixty-seven patients completed the PAID study in the pilot phase. The pilot study was performed to do the following:

1. Formulate the logistical and technical procedures and aspects involved in the clinical application of the instruments
2. Produce forms to facilitate the application of inferential statistics
3. Ensure the feasibility of the instruments
4. Demonstrate the usefulness of the instruments

Patients who came to medical attention with a wide variety of diagnoses were selected for recruitment to test the instruments and staff before initiation of the main study. This endeavor enabled modification of the instruments and in training of the clinical staff. It was determined that monetary incentives would have to be increased to attract the necessary number of patients for the study.

VALIDITY AND RELIABILITY STUDIES

After initial development of the PAI, the protocol was validated and tested for reliability. The main purpose of the reliability and validity phase was to fully validate the instruments that were revised after the pilot phase.

A multiphase process was used to develop, standardize, and validate the pain assessment protocol. The questionnaires for this study originated with the Pain Commission's suggestions for items or indicators hypothesized to be potentially helpful in pain assessment. A team of experts on chronic pain from around the country expanded on these initial items in the series of roundtable discussions. They included all areas of investigation thought necessary to produce a comprehensive list. The structure of the PAI is individual items combined into domains. The initial items and domains were based on the recommendations of the expert panel and literature review. They were modified by means of factor analysis. Individual items were grouped into similar categories or indices called *components*. Individual components were grouped to form the major *domains*. Each of these domains is tabulated with the component constructs in Table 3-1.

The three primary types of validity were assessed—concurrent, construct, and content. Each of these validation analyses is discussed separately. Reliability analyses were performed in this phase to ensure that the data were repeatable.

Table 3-1 Domains and Constructs

Domain	Construct
A. Rating of pain dimensions	Pain description Psychological perception of pain Perception of control over pain Pain behaviors Pain interference with sleep
B. Medical information	Use of health care Medication and tolerance of painful medical procedures Family history Physical examination findings Effectiveness of past treatments Review of diagnostic evaluations and procedures Review of medications, past and current
C. Mental health	Depression Emotional status Contact with the mental health system Substance abuse
D. Social support networks	Significant other support of person with pain
E. Functional limitations	Effect on concentration and cognitive processes Effect on activities of daily living Effect on emotional status Functional abilities
F. Employment or rehabilitation	Rehabilitation and work potential Motivation

A total of 651 patients completed the PAID study in the VCU—Medical College of Virginia (MCV) reliability and validity phase (Table 3-2). To perform the analyses, it was necessary to recruit both employed and unemployed persons on an equal basis. This was the only additional demographic constraint on this sample. Although no attempts were made to stratify the sample, it was found that women were slightly overrepresented, and the age and race distributions were comparable with the distribution in Virginia census statistics.

The main purpose of the national validity phase was to replicate the construct validation on a representative sample of Social Security disability applicants and to predict the pain and employment outcomes of the claimants. This was the predictive validity component of the study. The instruments were revised after the reliability and validity phase, and the final revisions were made after the national validity analyses were completed.

A total of 691 claimants completed the PAID study in the national validity phase. The sites were chosen to obtain a representative cross

Table 3-2 Demographic Composition of the Pain Assessment Instrument Validity Sample (n = 651)

Demographic Description	No. of Participants	Percentage
Race		
Black	189	29.0
White	438	67.3
Other	24	3.7
Sex		
Male	263	40.4
Female	388	59.6
Age (y)		
Younger than 40	280	43.0
40–54	303	46.5
55 and older	68	10.4

section of disability applicants. One site was chosen in each of six SSA regions. As it turned out, the chosen sites reflected the variation in the SSA disability determination process because some sites were SSA offices operating through the Vocational Rehabilitation system and others were not. Some sites were in decentralized states, whereas others covered the entire state. The sites were Indianapolis, Indiana; St. Louis, Missouri; Albuquerque, New Mexico; Philadelphia, Pennsylvania; Richmond, Virginia; and Seattle, Washington. The sample was stratified to be representative of the SSA claimant population for the demographic variables of sex, age, and ethnic origin.

The sample was divided equally among Social Security Disability Insurance (SSDI) applicants and Supplemental Security Income (SSI) or concurrent applicants. Because SSI applicants are not required to have worked previously and SSDI applicants must have a history of work to receive disability benefits, it was important that the sample represent both groups. Although all claimants within the study were identified as initial applicants, it was understood that some applicants may have applied before, and the case had been reopened. Claimants in all phases participated in 6- and 12-month follow-up interviews.

RESULTS

Reliability

Rater Reliability
Rater reliability was tested throughout the reliability and validity phase of the PAID project to ensure that the pain instruments and

Table 3-3   Rater Reliability Scores

Domain	Test-retest (same test administrator)	Interrater (different test administrator)
Patient perspective (total)	0.63	0.61
Rating of pain dimensions	0.62	0.58
Medical information	0.69	0.71
Mental health	0.71	0.62
Social support networks	0.51	0.48
Functional limitations	0.56	0.54
Physician perspective (total)	0.70	0.61
Rating of pain dimensions	0.83	0.75
Medical information	0.67	0.62
Mental health	0.79	0.52
Social support networks	0.74	0.50
Functional limitations	0.75	0.68

Cohen's κ and weighted Cohen's κ were used for all tests. All indices reached or exceeded target reliability rates.

methods of implementation provided consistent information. ***Rater reliability*** refers to the extent to which measurement error is created either by the implementation of a questionnaire from one time to another (test-retest reliability) or by implementation of the same instrument by a different administrator (interrater reliability) (Table 3-3). ***Test-retest reliability*** can be viewed as how closely the *same test administrator* agrees with earlier survey responses given by the same patient. ***Interrater reliability*** determines the extent to which *different test administrators* agree when giving the test to the same persons.

Twenty percent of the participating patients were randomly selected for a second recruitment to undergo the battery of assessments for reliability analyses. In the second assessment, care was taken to match patients with physicians and nurses who had assessed them previously and to mix patients with different sets of clinical researchers. A total of 99 patients were examined twice with two sets of instruments. The patients were chosen randomly and were demographically similar to the entire sample. The target time span of 3 weeks between assessments was exceeded slightly, the second assessment being completed an average of 31 days after the first. ***Cohen's κ rater reliability*** was used as a *highly conservative reliability statistic* that takes into account chance agreement. For variables with continuous or scaled (Likert) response options, a weighted Cohen's κ was used. Intraclass correlations were performed on a large percentage of the data as a comparative reliability statistic.

Highly variable items were dropped or combined until both test-retest reliability and interrater reliability for each instrument were reached.

Index Reliability

After the rater reliability analyses, index reliability was tested. **Index reliability** *is the extent to which each domain within each instrument and the constructs within the domains have internal consistency*. The index reliability was measured for all 651 patients. The components of the indices included the continuously scaled Likert response and appropriate yes-no response questions. For each domain and its specific constructs, an index was created within a specific instrument only if at least two scaled items represented the domain or construct within the instrument. A high index reliability ensures the use of such indices with confidence that the questions within the index are sufficiently related to each other. This allows analysis to be performed on the index rather than individual variables. Therefore, high index reliability indicates good internal consistency for the index in question.

Chronbach α item analysis *is the universally accepted statistic for index reliability*. This analysis was performed on each related group of questions, or index, within each of the instruments (for example, all the mental health questions on the form). The target rate for index reliability, called the α score, was an internal consistency of 0.70. Domains and constructs with lower index reliability were examined, and questions that appeared to be inconsistent with the others in the domain category were removed or placed into more appropriate domains.

All indices used in subsequent analyses reached or exceeded the target rate.

Validity

Concurrent Validity

Concurrent validity analyses were performed to determine whether the PAI measured specific circumstances in addition to previously validated tools (Table 3-4). Although it is generally acknowledged that pain is a multidimensional experience, there is currently no single comprehensive pain measurement instrument. There also are no instruments for the assessment of chronic pain that span the breadth of the PAID project instruments. Several standardized instruments that focus on specific aspects of the pain experience, or domains, were used to assess the concurrent validity of the PAID project instruments. Concurrent validity was obtained with the following commonly used, standardized, and validated instruments:

- Center for Epidemiological Studies Depression Scale (CES-D)
- Family Adaptability and Cohesion Evaluation Scale: Couple Version (FACES III)

Table 3-4 Concurrent Validity Analyses between Previously Validated Instruments and Related Indices of the Pain Assessment Instrument

Instrument	Index	n	Correlation Coefficient	Significance Level
CES-D	—	199	0.80	.0001
FACES III	Patient	56	0.31	.0204
	Significant other	51	0.60	.0001
MPI	Pain	129	0.73	.0001
	Interference	104	0.55	.0001
	Life control	133	0.41	.0001
	Affective distress	129	0.21	.0149
	Support	129	0.33	.0001
	Punishing responses	110	0.34	.0003
	Solicitous responses	129	0.51	.0001
	Distracting responses	129	0.42	.0001
	Household chores	108	0.62	.0001
	Outdoor work	109	0.23	.0158
	Activities from home	109	0.24	.0131
	Social activities	110	0.21	.0282
	General activity	133	0.34	.0001
MPQ	—	97	0.43	.0001
Oswestry	Functional limitations	117	0.71	.0001
	Sex	67	0.52	.0001
	Sleep	106	0.58	.0001
	Pain	104	0.42	.0001
	Activities of daily living	67	0.50	.0001
Waddell	—	55	0.67	.0001

Concurrent validity analyses assess whether the PAI measured specific areas in addition to previously validated or proved instruments.

CES-D, Center for Epidemiological Studies Depression Scale; FACES III, Family Adaptability and Cohesion Evaluation Scale: Couple Version; MPI, Multidimensional Pain Instrument; MPQ, McGill Pain Questionnaire.

- McGill Pain Questionnaire (MPQ)
- Multidimensional Pain Instrument (MPI)
- Oswestry, Shropshire low back pain assessment (Oswestry)
- Summary of Nonorganic Physical Signs in Low Back Pain (Waddell)

The concurrent validity phase of the study ensured three critical conditions: (1) that the instruments were tested with statistically appropriate groups; (2) that the PAI was demonstrated to have high correlation with reliable, valid, and currently used instruments in the field; and (3) that the instruments were usable in subsequent phases of the PAID project.

Construct Validity

Construct validity analyses *were performed to assess which domains and components actually were measured with the instrument.* Accurate measurement of construct validity is difficult, and factor analysis provides the most commonly used statistic of construct validity. However, if an inadequate sample is used, other factor combinations that adequately explain the variance in the data may be congruent with the one chosen with the analyzed sample. To confirm the adequacy of the PAID samples, Kaiser's measure of sampling adequacy (MSA) was performed on all factor samples.

Based on recommendations of the statistical panel, principal factor analysis with varimax rotation of factors was performed for each of the instruments on the items or selected indices that composed the domains. Selected indices comprise related questions within a group and are parts of components or domains. Items with high loading for a factor explain a component of variation for that factor. Before analysis, all scaled items were arranged from positive to negative (all items beginning with negative options were reversed). Questions related to claimants' experiences before the onset of pain were inappropriate for factor analysis because of the time frame and therefore were excluded from analysis.

Performing an independent analysis for each instrument has two main advantages. First, the instruments were designed to obtain the data from four unique perspectives, as follows:

- The claimant
- The person closest to the claimant*
- The claimant's regular or treating physician
- The consulting physician who has never examined the claimant

Comparison of these distinct perspectives, called methods, is in itself an indicator of validity.

Second, although they are distinct models, the instruments measure the same domains. For individual items, this would cause inflated correlations between items and produce deceptive or unreliable results in the factor analysis. Because of this, it is appropriate to combine the instruments for analysis on the domain level or on the construct level but not on the item level.

Although all generated factors were reviewed, only factors with eigen values of 1.0 or greater were retained in the final analysis. Significant factors were collected from each of the three assessment instruments relating to the claimant's pain: (1) the patient form (CSPI), (2) the treating physician form (PSPI-TP), and (3) the consulting physician

---

*A form collecting data from the claimant's significant other was tested and found to not contribute additional information or add to the reliability and validity of the PAI; therefore, it was deleted.

form (PSPI-CP). In the study, two physicians examined each patient and were designated *treating* or *consulting*. The forms were more detailed for treating than for consulting physicians. Twelve factors were retained by the factor analysis of the patient form. Six factors from the instrument for significant others (CSPI-SO) were retained. Eight factors were retained by the factor analysis of the treating physician form.

A corollary analysis of variance (ANOVA) and multitrait-multimethod (MTMM) analysis were completed on the same sample as a confirmation of the construct validity. Each domain (A through F) was considered a separate trait, and each of the four instruments was considered a different method. The ANOVA therefore compared each of the domains across the four forms as six different analyses. Student-Newman-Keuls post hoc means tests were performed for each of the five domains in which significant differences had been detected. The MTMM analysis compared the correlations across six traits and four methods (each of the four instruments) in a single analysis.

With these methods, analysis of the construct validity of the revised PAI succeeded in identifying the specific elements being measured with the PAI.

The *high level of agreement* between the two physician factor analyses (although the ANOVA determined the physician instruments to be separate models) supports the results of the analyses. ANOVA strengthens the use of these two separate instruments.

Content Validity

Content validity analyses were performed to measure the possibility of categorizing a person with respect to a specific variable (the criterion variable) by measuring other variables (predictor variables). ***Discriminant function analysis** is the primary statistical test used to discriminate between categories of a criterion variable, using several predictor variables.* If the criterion variable were to have a continuous distribution, such as age or weight, the test of choice would be multiple regression analysis. For predicting employment variables, such as salary, length of employment or unemployment, level of disability, or pain, on a scale, regression also would be the statistic of choice. This is necessary only when a continuous scale is to be measured or predicted. The ***discriminant function***, also called a *classification criterion, is created by generating a measure of generalized squared distance.* The distribution within each of the new groups created is approximately multivariate normal.

Discriminant analysis is similar to multiple regression in that both statistical techniques involve two or more predictor variables and a single criterion variable. Discriminant analysis, however, is limited to the special case in which the criterion is a person's group membership. In the discriminant analysis equation, a person's scores on the predictor variables are used in an attempt to predict the group of which the person is a member. In discriminant analysis equations, a weight, called a *discrimination function coefficient,* is applied to each applicant's score on each variable. The weights are similar to β weights in a multiple regression equation. The applicant's standard-ized score on the instruments' variables are multiplied by this weight to predict group membership at that point or at a later point in time, as with the PAID study.

The discriminant function coefficients do not indicate the magni-tude of correlation between each of the predictor variables and the crite-rion variable. A bivariate correlational statistic, such as product-moment *r* can be used to determine the degree of relation between each predictor variable and the criterion variable.

Previous research on predictors of return to work have produced predictor variables *inappropriate* for disability determination. Many have highlighted previous work history and demographic features such as age as the strongest predictors. Because it was believed that the SSA did not want to emphasize these characteristics in the deter-mination of disability, discriminant function analysis was performed without these variables. **Therefore, the predictor variables within this study, and for SSA purposes, are stronger in relation to the areas of an individual person's physical limitations and basic functional abil-ities than is the published body of research in chronic pain and meth-ods of predicting return to work.**

Content validity was analyzed with respect to three primary out-comes 6 months after assessment. Discriminant function analyses were performed on the subjective variables collected and were related to the patient's pain. The following specific outcomes were addressed:

1. The patient's potential for employment
2. The state of patient's future employment situation—same, better, or worse than at assessment
3. The level of intensity of pain—same, better, or worse than at assessment

The scoring of all items was based on the perceived contribution to the predictor equations indicated by the discriminant analyses. Therefore, each item that appeared to have a discriminant predictive value was assigned a weight based on its value in relation to the other items used. The results of the content validity analyses indicated that there were 60 to 65 highly discriminant variables for each of the three outcome variables. Because the content validity analyses were per-formed to test the subjective assessment of pain, basic demographic features such as age, race, sex, education, marital status, living situa-tion, employment history, and family medical history were not included in the analyses. It was anticipated that the predictor vari-ables would be the factors extracted from the principal factor analysis or the indices found to have a high reliability in the item analysis. The predictor equations obtained contained all variables that were found to have a significant unique contribution to one of the equations. The greatest discriminant difference between the analyses with the patient's significant other form and those without it was only 3%. Therefore, this form was deleted because the information obtained did not add significance to the predictive ability of the PAI.

The discriminant ability of the final set of predictors was considerably greater than chance for all three criterion variables, when the outcomes of the same set of patients were predicted 6 months after assessment.

Predictive Validity

Because the predictor variables in the content validity analyses demonstrated considerable discriminant ability for each of the three criterion variables, the next phase in the project was to ask: Do the instruments have predictive validity? That is, *Can it be predicted which persons within an SSA claimant population will or should return to work?* To answer these questions in the predictive validity analysis, the formulas from the content validity analyses were used. Predictive validity analysis requires a sample as structurally close as possible to the actual national SSA claimant population. The sample was stratified to be representative of the SSA claimant population for the demographic variables of sex, age, and ethnic origin.

The discriminant function formula obtained in the content validity phase was applied to predict the three criterion variables in the predictive validity sample. Although this is a discriminant function analysis, the result is called *predictive validity* rather than *content validity* because a formula is derived with one sample to predict a certain outcome for a separate sample. In the content validity phase, the formulas were applied to the sample with which they were created. Therefore, any unique variation in the sample, called error variation, would be expressed as an increase in predictive value of the formula. Applying these formulas to a second sample provides a predictive validation of the formulas. This process applies equally to regression and discriminant analysis, the main distinction being the nature of the criterion variable.

The content validity analyses provided empirical prediction of the claimant's situation 6 months after assessment. After implementation of the early reliability and validity phase, the research design was modified by SSA to be event driven. After the change, the follow-up interviews were based on application and decision dates rather than on assessment date. Therefore, two follow-up interviews were conducted in the predictive validity phase—one 6 months after application for disability and the other 6 months after the decision.

This report addresses only follow-up analyses conducted after decisions. It was anticipated, however, that the aforementioned change in design might have reduced the predictive value of the discriminant formulas generated in the early reliability and validity phase. Therefore, it also was likely that the content validity analyses would be repeated during the predictive validity phase. These newly generated formulas may be applied to a second SSA claimant sample during a field testing component of future research and development to further strengthen the formula with respect to this particular population.

Predictive Validity: Claimant Employed or Unemployed   Prediction of whether a claimant would be employed 6 months after a disability decision was considerably greater than chance with an overall prediction success rate of 90.2%. However, the ratio of employed persons to unemployed persons in the early validity phase (the VCU/MCV reliability and validity phase) was forced to be 1 to ascertain the characteristic differences between employed persons with chronic pain and unemployed persons with chronic pain. Because probabilities were used in the analysis and the predictive validity sample was so different from the earlier VCU/MCV sample for this criterion variable (only 13% of the national validity sample employed at follow-up interviews), the predictive ability of this equation was reduced the most, to 52.8%. This result was anticipated in the original research design. The constraint of a small sample size necessitated that there be a greater proportion of employed applicants in the early reliability and validity phase. The design specified repeat analyses during the subsequent SSA field test phase. Again, controlling the prior probabilities greatly increased the predictive validity of the formula.

Predictive Validity: Claimant's Change in Employment Situation
Changes in a claimant's employment situation could be predicted accurately 91.5% of the time in the early reliability and validity phase and 92.8% of the time in the predictive validity phase when the same sample was used. Because a small percentage of the claimants (approximately 10%) had a change in employment situation, the discriminant predictive validity will always appear high if proportional prior probabilities are used. It was originally anticipated that the discriminant ability of the predictor equation would be reduced to approximately 70%. The predictive ability of the equation generated from the VCU/MCV content validity analyses against the predictive validity sample actually was 76.1%, well within the anticipated range. Because it is unlikely that disability applicants would ever have an employment situation worsen between application or decision and follow-up evaluation, the inability of the equation to predict this occurrence is inconsequential and therefore was eliminated from the national validity analyses.

Predictive Validity: Claimant's Change in Pain Intensity   Although the discriminant ability of the formula regarding the change in claimant's pain intensity appears low (51.6% to 67.8% for predictions in the same sample), it is actually much greater than chance when the prior probabilities are considered. Approximately one third of claimants had improvement in pain, and approximately one third became worse, which makes discriminant predictive ability due to chance little more than 40%. This means, however, that the discriminant ability of the early content validity equation to predict a patient's pain situation in the future is not better than chance.

CONCLUSION

The instruments that compose the pain assessment instrument have been subjected to pilot study and validated. Construct validity analysis confirmed the existence of distinct domains related to pain. Concurrent validity analysis confirmed that the instruments measure the areas they were intended to measure when the component areas were comparatively measured with previously validated instruments. When the PAI was completed by trained personnel and the data collected were analyzed with the computerized equation, likelihood of return to work among a national population of SSA disability applicants with chronic pain was accurately predicted 87% of the time. In a general population with demographic features similar to those of Virginia, the prediction was accurate 90% of the time. This work was a major scientific achievement. It was given an A rating by the SSA, and the results have been published in the *Clinical Journal of Pain*, a peer-reviewed scientific journal.

Glossary of Statistical Terms

analysis of variance (ANOVA) A statistical technique that isolates and assesses the contribution of categorical independent variables to variation in the mean of a continuous dependent variable.

Chronbach's α item analysis The universally accepted statistic for index reliability.

Cohen's κ rater reliability A highly conservative reliability statistic that takes into account chance agreement.

concurrent validity The extent to which the index from one test correlates with that of a nonidentical test or index. Used to predict performance in a real-life situation at about the same time as the test or procedure.

construct validity The extent to which a test or procedure appears to measure a higher order, inferred theoretical construct, or trait in contrast to measuring a more limited, specific dimension.

content validity The extent to which the items of a test or procedure are a representative sample of that which is to be measured.

discriminant function analysis The primary statistical method used to discriminate between categories of a criterion variable using several predictor variables.

eigen value A scalar associated with a given linear transformation of a vector phase and having the property that there is a nonzero vector which when multiplied by the scalar is equal to the vector obtained by letting the transformation operate on the vector.

index reliability The extent to which each of the domains within each of the instruments and the constructs within the domains have internal consistency. For each domain and its specific constructs, an index is created within a specific instrument only if at least two scaled items represent the domain or construct within the instrument. High index reliability ensures the use of such indices with confidence that the questions within the index are sufficiently related to each other and allows analyses to be performed on the index rather than individual variables. High index reliability indicates good internal consistency for the index in question.

interrater reliability The extent to which different test administrators agree when administering a test to the same persons.

Kaiser's measure of sampling adequacy (MSA) Analysis used to determine the adequacy of the sample tested.

predictive validity The extent to which performance can be predicted in a real-life task at a future time.

rater reliability The extent to which measurement error is created either by the implementation of a questionnaire from one time to another or by implementation of the same instrument by a different administrator.

test-retest reliability The extent to which the same test administrator agrees with earlier survey responses provided by the same patient.

4 Content of the Pain Assessment Instrument

PAIN SCREENING INSTRUMENT

The Pain Screening Instrument (PSI) is a questionnaire that was conceptualized in the Pain Assessment Instrument Development (PAID) study to be administered to all claimants when they applied for SSA disability benefits. Use of this instrument standardized the assessment of pain and helped identify the complaint of pain for disability applicants across all recipient categories. The PSI contains 10 items that are the most indicative of pain, and information comes entirely from the respondent's (pain claimant's) viewpoint. It must be emphasized, however, that because the PSI was created as a result of this research, it was not independently validated at the culmination of this research project. Within the original design, it was anticipated that this screening instrument would undergo validation during a field-testing phase within the Social Security Administration (SSA). The nature of this instrument required that it be administered at the time of application for disability, which means that the PSI would not be used by the SSA until the instruments had undergone extensive field testing within the SSA disability determination process. As part of the Pain Assessment Instrument (PAI), the PSI can be used as a short form to identify the complaint of 6 months of pain and used for screening for appropriateness of a patient for a chronic pain program. The PSI does not have to be used or completed, but it is included in this book because it may be useful in some practices (see Appendix 1).

PATIENT ASSESSMENT INSTRUMENT

The Patient Assessment is a questionnaire used to assess the patient's perception of the following: history, location, frequency, duration, severity, and intensity of pain with exacerbating factors; history of use of health care for diagnosis and management of pain (e.g., surgical, pharmaceutical, physician visits, hospitalizations); current use of and future need for health care; pain behaviors before and since onset of pain; cognitive status and ability for task completion; emotional disturbance before and since the onset of pain; history of mental health intervention; activities of daily living (ADL); social functioning before and since the onset of pain; and functional ability and limitations (see Appendix 2).

PHYSICIAN ASSESSMENT INSTRUMENT

The Physician Assessment is a questionnaire and examination form used by a physician to evaluate the following patient-claimant characteristics: description of pain, including sensory and affective intensity; frequency and duration of pain; use of health care systems; exhibition of pain behaviors; emotional status; cognitive and functional status; ability to complete a task; physical examination and evidence of physical impairment; laboratory and imaging data to support the patient's description of pain; and functional ability and rehabilitation potential. The form also has a historical section that outlines previous services, treatments, and medications (see Appendix 3).

In the PAID study, two physician forms were used to collect data—the physician assessment instrument (see Appendix 3) and a shorter version, the consulting physician form. The study results did not justify two distinct physician instruments. Nevertheless, the protocol design, when used to predict return to work, requires evaluations by two physicians; therefore, a Physician Assessment Instrument is completed by both. When completing the Integrated Pain Report (IPR), one will be referred to as the treating physician (TP) and the other as the consulting physician (CP).

INTEGRATED PAIN REPORT

The IPR consists of individual items combined into domains. The structure is hierarchical in nature with comprehensive domains. This structure is the culmination of the statistical analyses conducted in the study, specifically the construct validity factor analysis and the discriminant function analyses. Individual items are completed across the respective forms, grouped into similar categories or indices, and called components. Individual components are grouped to form the six major domains to produce a concise IPR, which can be easily interpreted for consideration of the individual patient or claimant.

In the PAID study, all data for each claimant with chronic pain were merged to produce the domains of the IPR for this person. Weights for each item on the IPR were based on the predictive value of each item. These were obtained from the discriminant validity analyses. A claimant profile was created with the IPR, and a prediction whether the person would return to work within 6 months was computed. Only valid and reliable items from the instruments were included in the final products (see Appendix 4).

PAIN DOMAINS

The structure of the instruments consists of individual items combined into domains (see Table 3-1). These initial items and domains were based on findings of a review by an expert panel and of a literature review. The present structure is more hierarchical in nature, having fewer, more comprehensive domains. Individual items are completed across the respective forms and grouped into components. Individual components are grouped to form the six major domains. The domains and components of the domains are as follows:

    A. **Rating of pain dimensions.** Includes pain description items such as frequency, length, intensity, and unpleasantness; psychological perception of pain, pain behaviors, and perception of control over pain; and interference with sleep. Information is collected through patient reports and physician ratings.

    B. **Medical information.** Includes use of health care, use of medication, willingness to tolerate painful medical procedures, results of diagnostic tests, diagnosis, cause of pain, and answers to a series of questions related to the physical examination performed by physicians. Collected through patient reports and physician ratings.

    C. **Mental health status.** Includes the patient's self-report of depressive symptoms, contact with the mental health system, substance abuse, and sociopathy; significant other's perception of substance abuse; and physicians' perceptions of depression, substance abuse, and other mental health indicators.

    D. **Social support networks.** Includes the patient's perception of support provided by significant other, the patient's perception of the significant other's reaction to the patient, and each physician's perception of the patient's social support network.

    E. **Functional limitations.** Includes assessment of the effect of pain on concentration, cognitive processes, and ADL, and emotional status and functional abilities perceived by the patient and physicians. This domain has been broken into two domains:

        a. *Functional limitations and ADL.* Includes assessment of the effect of pain on the claimant's concentration and cognitive processes, ADL, and emotional status as it relates to function perceived by the claimant

        b. *Functional abilities.* Includes assessment of functional abilities of the claimant perceived primarily by physicians.

    F. **Employment or rehabilitation potential.** Includes, for the purposes of the construct and content validity analyses, the perceptions of physicians regarding the patient's employment potential and motivation to work.

Not all forms contain every domain, and the emphasis within some domains changes between forms. Each domain can be broken into components that are indices of related variables within a domain. All items on each of the instruments refer to the claimant-patient and often are the respondent's perception of how an action affects the claimant-patient. The analyses were performed on the aforementioned domains and on the items that compose each of the individual instruments.

5 Administration and Utilization of the Pain Assessment Instrument

---

HOW TO USE THE PAIN ASSESSMENT INSTRUMENT

This chapter contains information to assist clinicians in completing the data forms. Included are parameters for range of motion and various definitions. The following steps are recommended for implementation of the Pain Assessment Instrument (PAI) in the clinical setting:

1. Read through each question on the physician instrument and on the patient instrument. This enables the clinician to become familiar with the information being collected from both the physician's perspective and the patient's perspective.

2. Read this chapter completely. The parameters and definitions provided must be used to ensure consistent and reliable completion of the forms.

3. Allow extra time in your schedule for the first five or six patients who will use the PAI. Until clinicians become familiar with the data needed to complete the forms, it will take longer to collect this information. As clinicians become more familiar with them, the instruments can then be completed in an almost consistent amount of time. Patients differ in ability to respond efficiently to questions, and this must be taken into account in scheduling. In the beginning, the process of collecting the data and entering them onto the form may seem burdensome, but it quickly becomes efficient if performed consistently and frequently.

4. Complete the forms as soon as possible after seeing the patient. The best time is immediately after the visit but before the patient leaves the room, in case a specific data element was not obtained. Waiting until after the patient leaves the office or later in the day may impair the accuracy and completeness of the information. Some clinicians may need someone in the office to assist them in assuring the forms are complete. The assistant can review the form as soon as the patient has been seen and follow up immediately with the clinician regarding any incomplete or missing information.

5.   Ensure that clinical assistants assigned to overseeing completion of the patient instrument become familiar with the form and with the dos and don'ts in completing the form. The assistant also needs to be aware of other questions that may be asked and be prepared to respond to pain behaviors (see pp. 54–55).

6.   Identify a method of keeping the forms separate from other patient files. This can be a separate place in the patient's chart or a separate file. Whether the completed PAI is considered part of the patient's formal medical record also has to be determined.

7.   Because this manual does not yet have accompanying software, the clinician may want to have the data from the Integrated Pain Report (IPR) entered onto software that is capable of transferring the collected information into a graph.

8.   Do not ask the patient for the information by reading or restating the questions on the Physician Assessment Instrument. The wording of the questions on the physician form is similar to that on the patient form. This information has already been collected from the patient; obtaining the data by restating the question verbatim only duplicates the patient's response, which you already have.

INSTRUMENT COMPLETION TIME

A great deal of variability exists in the amount of time it takes to complete the instruments. During the national validity phase, claimants took an average of 55 minutes to complete the patient form, although the standard deviation was 21 minutes. Whereas the measures of central tendency were fairly equivalent (mean 55 minutes, median 50 minutes, mode 55 minutes), the distribution curve was fairly flat. Several claimants completed the instrument quickly, and others took as long as 2 hours. It is projected that the time for completion can be reduced, but some patients always will need additional time and assistance with the instrument depending on educational level, intelligence quotient, presence of language barriers, and similar factors.

The time needed to complete the physician forms in the national phase was considerably shorter than that for the patient instrument. The average time was 28 minutes for the treating physician and 25 minutes for the consulting physician. In the study, two physicians assessed each patient independently. One form was the full physician form, and the physician functioned as if he or she were the patient's treating physician and knew the patient from previous visits. The second form was shorter, and the physician functioned as a consulting physician, the patient being new to the physician. In the Pain Assessment Instrument Development (PAID) study, almost all of the patients were unknown to both physicians, which increased completion time for the treating physician. The PAID study results did not justify two distinct physician instruments. When the protocol design is used to predict return to work calculated by using the computerized equation, the physician assessment instrument must be completed by two different physicians. They are designated as the treating physician (TP) and the consulting physician (CP) on the IPR.

This manual was designed for actual practice. The original PAI was designed as a research tool. This version of the PAI requires only one physician to complete the treating physician form because prediction of return to work will not be calculated. The final versions of the physician instruments with the history interview and examination take 20 to 25 minutes to complete (once the physician is familiar and comfortable with the forms and the parameters). To obtain the information necessary to complete the instruments accurately, the clinician must obtain a complete history and perform a complete physical examination. It is expected, however, that physicians completing the form will be familiar with the instrument and that a concise pain history and physical examination will be appropriate. First time users will need additional time.

PARAMETERS AND GUIDELINES FOR PHYSICIANS

SLEEP DISTURBANCES

Part I, Question 11 Has the patient reported sleep disturbances?

There are two primary aspects to this question. First, it is important to note whether the patient volunteers information about sleep patterns or needs to be asked. Given the prevalence of sleep disturbances among persons with chronic pain, it is recommended that patients be asked consistently about sleep patterns. For example, the physician may ask, "Are you experiencing any difficulties sleeping?"

The second aspect of this question involves the definition of a sleep disturbance. Sleep disorders often occur in conjunction with psychiatric disorders and with physical conditions that disrupt sleep. Sleep disorders are categorized into the following two subclasses:

A. **Parasomnia**—a disturbance in which an abnormal event occurs during sleep; includes night terrors, sleep-walking, and dream anxiety (nightmares).
B. **Dyssomnia**—disruption in amount, quantity, or quality of sleep; there are three categories: insomnia, hypersomnia, and sleep-wake schedule disorders. Insomnia is the most common type of dyssomnia and can occur at different times, as follows:
   - *Sleep-onset insomnia*—difficulty falling asleep on the first attempt to sleep in the evening
   - *Inability to maintain sleep*—waking frequently throughout the night and being unable to sustain sleep for more than 2 to 3 hours at a time

- *Early morning awakening*—sleep disorder most frequently associated with depression

Nonrestorative sleep is another area of dyssomnia with or without sleep-onset insomnia or difficulty maintaining sleep. It is commonly attributed to and caused by chronic pain. Sleep disturbances usually impair daytime functioning and cause irritability and fatigue. Patients with chronic pain generally report sleep-onset insomnia, frequent awakening,[50] and nonrestorative sleep.[51,52] Early morning awakening is reported but less frequently than the other disorders.

For the purpose of this instrument, sleep disturbance is defined according to *Diagnostic and Statistical Manual of Mental Disorders, Fourth Edition,* criteria. As a routine part of the examination, the physician should identify how a patient is generally sleeping. If the patient reports difficulty with sleep, it is important to ascertain what type of sleep problems are experienced, such as sleep-onset insomnia, early morning awakening, frequent nighttime awakening, or nonrestorative sleep. A sleep problem that occurs more than 2 times a week for longer than 1 month meets the diagnostic criteria of a sleep disorder.

RANGE OF MOTION

Part I, Question 15 Abnormalities in Range of Motion

Abnormal range of motion is assessed according to functional effect and degrees of loss of motion. Normal changes associated with aging must be considered. For example, for a 60-year-old person, a loss of 10 degrees of rotation in cervical range of motion would be considered a normal effect of aging. A 10-degree decrease in cervical rotation at any age would have little functional impact. However, with loss of only a few degrees of range of motion of one of the fingers or the thumb, function would be greatly impaired. Because of these variations, definition of the parameters used is important (Table 5-1). It allows age-appropriate determination of loss of range of motion and the significance of the loss to the patient.

Table 5-1   Parameters of Range of Motion

Answer	Definition
None	Normal or appropriate for age
Slight	Mild loss of motion (less than 15% of total) or loss of motion with minimal clinical significance
Moderate	Loss of motion, up to 50%; clinically significant
Marked	Loss of 50% or more loss of motion in major joint; clinically significant
Extreme or rigid	No motion or jog of motion in major joint

DIAGNOSTIC TESTS SUPPORTING PAIN COMPLAINT

> **Part I, Question 26** How much support do laboratory studies give to the patient's reports?

Support implies that a given diagnostic test provides additional objective evidence to substantiate the diagnosis the clinician has based on the patient's history and clinical examination findings.

Degree of Support

To gauge the degree of support offered by a given diagnostic test for a given medical condition (e.g., mild, moderate, strong, unequivocal, or not supportive) depends on a given physician's knowledge, anecdotal experience, bias, and reasoning ability. The answer to this question can vary from diagnosis to diagnosis, physician to physician. The most reasonable consensus may be gained from encouraging physicians to answer this question on the basis of common practice and confirmation from reports of well-controlled studies.

Abnormal versus Normal Findings

Concern may arise about whether the concept of support should be limited to diagnostic tests with abnormal findings only. It appears clear that we typically use normal findings from diagnostic tests to derive a diagnosis by means of exclusion. However, it complicates this question to do so because any study performed can be argued to be supportive of a diagnosis. In the interest in simplicity, *only abnormal findings should be entertained as potentially supportive of a diagnosis.*

Normal findings are *not* considered supportive regardless of the diagnosis. For example, fibromyalgia as an isolated medical problem is not associated with abnormal findings of imaging or laboratory studies. It can be argued, therefore, that normal findings of laboratory tests "support" the diagnosis. For the sake of optimizing consensus among examining physicians, the presence of conditions such as fibromyalgia, which characteristically lack abnormal findings at diagnostic testing is *not* considered supported by normal test results.

ESTIMATING PATIENT EFFORT

> **Part II, Question 8** In your estimation, what level of effort will the patient expend if a functional capacity evaluation is performed?

Effort exerted by a patient during a functional capacity evaluation (FCE) is determined by measuring the consistency of strength measurements (reproducibility of hand grip dynamometer testing). In estimating the level of effort a patient expends on an FCE, the physician should be aware of and be able to assess the following:

1. **Consistency of motion and muscle testing at physical examination.** For example, a patient with 5% forward flexion at spinal range of motion testing who bends over to take off his

socks is unlikely to have consistent or maximal effort in an FCE.

2. **Attitude and personality of patient.** Patients who want to be "good patients" and please the physician or those who have compulsive perfectionist tendencies may exert extreme effort in an FCE. This can be misleading because they are unlikely to be able to sustain the effort for hours or days.

3. **Fear of reinjury or worsening of an injury that causes pain.** This usually results in sub maximum effort.

4. **Fear that health care professionals do not believe the patient has pain or do not understand the severity.** This causes the patient to exert submaximal effort to emphasize the effect of pain on function.

5. **Patient's level of knowledge.** Patients educated in body mechanics and ergonomics related to their pain may exert more realistic effort.

HEALTH CARE UTILIZATION

> **Part III, Question 10** To what degree has the patient used health care services compared with use by patients with similar problems?

When a patient is new to a clinician, there often are no data to define this variable. All available records should be reviewed, and the patient should be asked about other health services used. A judgment must be made to assess whether there is excessive use of health care. Specific clues may be multiple changes of physician or multiple evaluations by alternative medicine practitioners.

PATIENT COMPLIANCE

> **Part III, Question 11** To what degree has the patient been compliant with prescribed care?

When the literature was reviewed for study in 1991, no data were available for defining this variable. All patient records should be thoroughly reviewed to document compliance; examples are physical therapy records, which usually document the number of appointments kept and compliance with exercise. Patients can be asked about medicines that have been tried and why they failed and about who initiated discontinuation of the drug, the physician or the patient. If the patient is new to the physician, there may be no other means to assess compliance other than *impressions* from the physical examination and history.

EXCESSIVE PROCEDURES

> **Part III, Question 12** To what degree has the patient expressed desire to undergo repeated painful diagnostic procedures or surgical treatment?

A history of undergoing repeated painful diagnostic procedures or operations (three or more) is considered evidence of excessive willingness. If there is no history of repeated surgical procedures, the patient should be asked the following: "If surgery had a 50% chance of making you better and a 50% chance of making you worse, would you undergo it?" The response will help grade the answer.

COPING AND DOCUMENTED IMPAIRMENT

> **Part IV, Question 1** Which of the following definitions best describe the patient's pain situation?
>
> No chronic pain.
> Chronic pain; inability to cope; insufficient documented impairment.
> Chronic pain; competent coping; insufficient documented impairment.
> Chronic pain; inability to cope; sufficient documented impairment.
> Chronic pain; competent coping; sufficient documented impairment.

Inability to Cope

Inability to cope can be defined as a patient who displays at least *two* of the following criteria:

1. **Prominent complaint of pain**—Assessed according to the *patient's perception* of the intensity of pain, not how much the patient vocalizes to the physician or family
2. **Psychological changes**—May be present alone or in combination; can include depression, increased dependency, anxiety, irritability, intolerance, hostility, fatigue, frustration, hopelessness, helplessness, or a decrease in attention span
3. **Employment problems**—Loss of employment, decrease in work productivity, or disruption of interpersonal relations in the work environment related to pain, as opposed to economic factors

and at least *one* of the following criteria:

1. **Drug-seeking behavior**
2. **Decrease in social activity attributable to pain behavior**
3. **Deterioration in ability to perform activities of daily living**
4. **Disruption of family dynamics attributable to pain behavior,** such as divorce, separation, child or spousal abuse, overdependency, and other changes consistent with family discord
5. **Overuse of medical care system,** such as multiple physician visits or multiple operations for the same condition, repeated courses of medicinal, physical, or occupational therapy despite minimal or no improvement

Documentation of Impairment

Impairment can be defined as a medically determinable physical or mental condition that can be expected to produce pain. This determination is based on common practice by physicians familiar with the diagnosis and management of a given medical condition. When clarification of specific impairment is necessary, determination can be supplemented with the American Medical Association *Guides to the Evaluation of Permanent Impairment*.[4]

Sufficient Documentation

Sufficient documentation can be defined as an indication that objective findings, measured and recorded with diagnostic tests or a clinical examination, are available for a given patient. *Sufficient documentation* should be interpreted to mean that objective findings are accurate and complete enough to support the presence of impairment, as determined by common practice and with AMA guidelines.[4]

Insufficient Documentation

Insufficient documentation occurs in instances in which diagnostic tests or examinations were never performed, were performed but the results are not available for review, or were performed but the results did not support impairment or were interpreted incorrectly. There is a complicating factor intrinsic to this issue. Patients given different diagnoses by different physicians may be given different interpretations of sufficient documentation. This may not mean a lack of reliability regarding the understanding of sufficiently documented impairment but may reflect the lack of diagnostic reliability in the patient's case.

EXAGGERATION AND MAGNIFICATION OF SYMPTOMS

> **Part IV, Question 2**   Did the patient react appropriately to the examination, or did the pain behaviors appear exaggerated?

Through clinical use Waddell et al.[39] standardized a group of five types of nonorganic physical signs of low back pain—tenderness, simulation tests, distraction, regional disturbance, and overreaction. Isolated positive results are discounted. *Three or more positive results* are strong evidence of magnification of symptoms and pain behaviors. These nonorganic signs are separable from and independent of the standard physical findings of organic pathologic conditions (see Chapter 2).

ASSESSING MOTIVATION TO WORK

> **Part IV, Question 5**   How motivated do you believe this patient has been or would be in terms of changing his or her lifestyle to be rehabilitated, for example, accept lower pay, move, or take a less desirable job?

Motivation must be judged in an overall sense during evaluation. If the patient has already made substantial lifestyle changes, it may be difficult to determine whether he or she is truly unwilling or willing to make additional changes for rehabilitation. Suggested questions include the following: "What jobs have you considered that may be more suitable because of the pain?" "Would you be willing to work a less desirable shift to be able to work?" and "Would you be willing to take a lower-grade job than you previously held? Willing to accept less pay? Willing to take a bus to a more distant job to be able to work?"

CORRELATION OF PAIN COMPLAINT WITH CLINICAL FINDINGS

> **Part IV, Question 6** To what extent are the descriptions of pain greater than would be expected from objective clinical findings?

Objective clinical findings can be defined as the correlation of history, physical examination findings, and results of diagnostic tests. A patient who has fibromyalgia, is found to have multiple tender and trigger points, and has altered his or her lifestyle because of pain would be expected to report less pain than a patient with the same diagnosis but who continues the same social and family obligations. A patient who believes that experiencing pain signals will worsen the injury or cause "something bad" to happen likewise may be expected to rate greater pain than one who expects to have pain because of age and wear and tear on the body. Therefore, the extent of pain reported (illness behavior) is compared with the pain expected because of the clinical diagnosis.

Dos and Don'ts

Throughout the Physician Assessment Instrument there are questions about the physician's "educated opinion" about the patient's pain, the patient's functional abilities, and the patient's social life. This line of questioning stems from the assertion that the physician learns a great deal about a patient during their interaction and physical examination. Using the strategies and guidelines provided in this chapter, answer the questions using your best judgement. The most extensive concentration of these questions is in Part III, Social Functioning and Development. The instructions state: "Please respond to the following questions based on your perceptions about and interactions with the patient." Do not ask the patient to provide this information. *Do not repeat the questions as worded on the form when questioning the patient.* The patient has already responded to the questions on the Patient Assessment Instrument. To repeat the question verbatim will only obtain the patient's subjective report, which you already have.

As you evaluate for signs of malingering or exaggerated symptoms, observe the patient to detect affect, or mood. A simple "How are things?" can release a wealth of information. The questions are interrelated. If a patient volunteers information about a recent social or sports event, for example, you may have sufficient information to answer several questions, such as questions 5, 15, 16, 17, and 19 in Part III (leisure activities, exercise, travel). An account of a recent interpersonal interaction may give you insight into the answer to questions 25 or 26.

Do ask open-ended and specific questions about activities of daily living to complete the functional abilities section. For example, ask, "Who does the grocery shopping?" That the patient shops alone may indicate he or she can push a cart, bend to pick up objects from lower shelves, or reach to obtain objects from higher shelves. Specific activity-related questions, such as whether the patient unloads the groceries and puts them away, will provide the same kind of information. Can the patient pick up a 2-liter bottle of soda or a 1-gallon jug of milk? Does the patient do house maintenance or change light bulbs in ceiling fixtures (indicating repetitive rotation above head)? Who cooks? Cooking requires lifting of heavy objects from below waist height to slightly above waist height and obtaining materials from overhead. Do determine whether the patient can perform these activities regularly or only sporadically. Don't ask the patient questions verbatim from the functional abilities form.

Do complete the form while in the office with the patient or at least before the patient leaves the office. Familiarity with the instrument will allow you to obtain all the necessary information during the history and examination processes without going question by question on the form. Do review the parameters section occasionally and keep a copy of the ROM parameter handy. If the PAI is used inconsistently and unregularly, review this chapter and the physician instrument before seeing the patient. Don't leave any questions unanswered. Do respond consistently to pain behavior by using the three-step response to pain behavior discussed later in this chapter.

Questions Patients May Ask Physicians

Why do you need this information?
Some patients may be suspicious that you are trying to determine whether they are faking. Most patients, however, appreciate the comprehensive approach to the problem.

Does this mean you think the problem is all in my head?
The patient needs to be reassured that there is no suggestion that the pain is not real or is "all in your head." This is a routine way to obtain complete information about pain and persons with pain to assist with evaluation and treatment.

Will this information be available to insurance companies, disability determiners, or lawyers?
If the completed forms are in the patient's chart, the information is considered part of the patient record and therefore is subject to the same access as the patient record. If the information is entered into a separate database, this may not be the case. Physicians should contact their attorneys for the answer to this question.

How to Respond to Pain Behaviors
Chapter 2 defines pain behaviors and discusses interpretation. Physicians and support staff should maintain a consistent response to pain behaviors. If there are variable responses, the ability to obtain reliable, consistent data may be impaired. When a patient states he or she can-

not perform a movement or assume a position required for physical examination and another position is not adequate to evaluate the patient, the following three steps are recommended:

> **Three-Step Response to Pain Behavior** This is a three-step method that should be done in the specified order:
> 1. "Cheerleading" approach
> 2. "It's necessary" approach
> 3. Stopping on the third refusal

1. Encourage the patient gently to try the position. Tell the patient that you are aware of the pain, you will do only what is necessary to evaluate them, and you will be as gentle as possible.
2. If the patient refuses, tell him or her that the examination must be complete for the best evaluation and treatment.
3. If the patient continues to refuse, eliminate that portion of the examination and record why the examination was incomplete.

TRAINING OF SUPPORT STAFF

Several support staff should be chosen, oriented, and trained in administration of the form. Patients are encouraged to complete the form themselves. Many patients have questions, some may not be able to read, and still others may need physical help to complete the form. Patients also may say they are in too much pain to complete the form. They should be allowed and encouraged to change position, such as sitting to standing, if this will help. The aforementioned three-step approach should be tried three times unless the patient says he or she must stop and cannot go on after the three attempts at cheerleading. If this occurs, the patient should be allowed to stop, and the staff member should offer to complete the form for the patient. This entails reading the question to the patient, reading the answer options, and checking the answer given by the patient. The support person should be sympathetic to the patient's condition and pain, but in no way should the staff member influence how the patient answers a question or give an opinion about the patient's answer.

The support staff must understand that it is crucial that all questions be answered. Every form should be reviewed for completeness before the patient leaves the office. If a patient does leave and the form is later found incomplete, the staff member can telephone the patient to ask the question. This must be done within 48 hours of the visit. The best approach, however, is to have the forms completed before the patient leaves the building.

The support staff should review the physician form before the patient and the physician leave and strongly encourage the physician to answer every question on the form. Sometimes this is difficult for busy physicians, but a persistent and effective support staff can make the difference in completing the database. The physician may want to leave the building, but the support staff should be instructed to mark the question that needs an answer, turn the form to that page, and follow the physician out of the office, if needed, to get the form completed.

SUGGESTED RESPONSES FOR SUPPORT STAFF WHEN CLARIFICATION IS REQUESTED

Frequently Asked Questions

From the Pain Screening Instrument

> **Questions 5a and 5b**   Please note the amount of unpleasantness your pain has caused you at the following levels:
> Usual intensity in the past week
> Highest intensity in the past week

Intensity also can be referred to as the strength of the pain, asking the patient, "How strong is the pain?"

From the Patient Assessment, Part I

> **Question 5**   History of Pain

Instruct the patient to include when the pain started.

> **Question 6**   Does the pain radiate to other areas?

Radiation can be defined as pain or an unpleasant sensation that moves from a central location such as the neck, shoulder, or back into a more peripheral location such as the arm, hand, or leg.

> **Question 10**   If you have had pain-free periods in the past 6 months, how long do they usually last?

Can be restated as, "Do you usually go months, weeks, or days without pain?"

> **Question 13b**   In the past 6 months, how many times have you seen a physician or health specialist for pain?

Health specialist can be defined as a physical or occupational therapist, nurse, or physician.

> **Question 17**   How much does the pain interfere with what you want to do? No restrictions? Minor interference? Moderate obstacle? Great barrier? Hindrance to all activity?

Pain as a moderate obstacle would frequently prevent the patient from achieving a desired action or outcome. Pain as a great barrier would almost always prevent the patient from accomplishing goals.

Question 19 Indicate the intensity of painful sensation when your pain was at the following levels.

Intensity of painful sensation can be defined to the patient as strength of pain.

Question 21c Has your significant other been supportive or helpful when you are in pain?

A significant other can be simply defined as a person in the patient's life who is the main emotional or physical support for him or her.

Question 21h Have you had disagreements with or avoided other family members?

It may be helpful to break this into two separate questions. "Have you had disagreements with other family members?" "Have you avoided other family members?"

Question 28a Have you ever had a period of self-imposed abstinence?

Abstinence can be simply defined as refraining from drinking, as doing without voluntarily.

Question 29 How often do you use recreational drugs?

Recreational drugs can be explained as those that are not for a medical problem, such as marijuana and cocaine.

Question 33d On the average, do the medicines you take always take the pain away? Always make the pain less? Usually take the pain away? Usually make the pain less? Provide little or no relief?

To simplify, this question can be restated as "Do the medications take the pain away or decrease the pain?" Then ask, "Usually or always?"

Question 34 In the past 6 months, how frequently and severely did you feel depressed, frustrated, anxious, angry, or guilty?

To differentiate *frequently* and *severely*, it is helpful to have the patient rate the frequency first (number of times) and then rate the severity (level of feeling).

From Patient Assessment, Part II: Medical Information

Questions 1–11 Before the pain, how often did you . . . ?
In the past 6 months, how often did you . . . ?

It may be helpful to have the patient answer the questions in relation to "before the pain" and then answer the questions in relation to "in the past 6 months."

From Patient Assessment, Part III

Question 1h   Have you ever had a myelogram for this problem?

A myelogram can be explained simply as an x-ray of the spinal cord in which contrast medium is inserted.

6 Predicting Subsequent Employment Status of SSA Disability Applicants with Chronic Pain

Karen S. Rucker, M.D., and Helen M. Metzler, M.S.*

This article is reprinted for the purposes of providing manual users with resources regarding validity of PAI. The MMPAP in this chapter is referred to as the PAI elsewhere in this manual.

ABSTRACT

Objective

The study assessed the predictive ability of the standardized Multi-perspective Multidimensional Pain Assessment Protocol (MMPAP). An assessment tool that predicts return to work with chronic pain patients is needed, as increasing numbers of disability applications are adjudicated in the courts.

Design

National randomized validation sample of disability applicants. Each MMPAP consisted of physical examinations by two physiatrists and the

*Reprinted with permission from KS Rucker and HM Metzler. Predicting subsequent employment status of SSA disability applicants with chronic pain. *Clin J Pain* 1995;11: 22–35.

Manuscript submitted June 9, 1994; first revision received September 15, 1994; second revision received November 8, 1994; accepted for publication November 22, 1994.

This work was sponsored by the Social Security Administration under contract no. 600-90-0229. Additional support was provided by two of the National Institutes of Health General Clinical Research Centers at Virginia Commonwealth University/ Medical College of Virginia (VCU/MCV) and the University of New Mexico (UNM). VCU/MCV is funded under NCRR grant M01 RR 00065. UNM is funded under NCRR grant 5M01 RR 00997-17.

participant's subjective assessment. Criterion standards were Multi-dimensional Pain Inventory and McGill Pain Questionnaire. There was phone follow-up 6 months postdecision.

Setting
Six clinical sites were ambulatory referral centers, both public and private.

Participants
Population-based random national sample of 710 Social Security disability applicants claiming chronic pain related to their disability, stratified by national Social Security Administration (SSA) applicant demographics. Seventy-eight were lost to follow-up, and 688 initially refused.

Interventions
No interventions were continued or initiated by the research team between assessment and follow-up.

Main Outcome Measures
Claimant employment status 6 months after disability decision was primary outcome, change in pain intensity, and change in employment situation.

Results
The MMPAP predicted with 90% accuracy employment status of SSA disability applicants with chronic pain 6 months postdecision when assessed at application by two physicians trained in physical medicine and rehabilitation (physiatry). Accuracy of employment situation change was 93%, and of pain intensity change was 65%. Self-report measures, physical examination results, psychological status, functional limitations, and physician's subjective appraisal predict future employment.

Conclusions
The MMPAP accurately predicts future employment of disability applicants claiming chronic pain. The introduction of this standardized protocol will assist in standardizing disability determination for claimants with chronic pain.

Key Words
Chronic pain, disability, employment

INTRODUCTION

The inability to perform work or to meet other adult role expectations (e.g., homemaker, parent, or spouse) due to chronic pain represents a large and growing problem. Functional impairment due to severe pain disrupts the lives of thousands of individuals each year, challenges the nation's health care system, and confounds the disability determination process. In a recent poll of Americans concerning their experience with severe pain, nearly one quarter of adults said that they experience pain strong enough to interfere with their daily activities a couple of times each month.[1] It has been estimated that pain causes more than $55 billion per year in lost workdays.[3]

The identification of pain as a component of disability has profound implications for public and private health care. For example, applications for Social Security Disability benefits increased by more than 40% in 1992.[54] In 1992, disability income maintenance programs such as Supplemental Security Income (SSI) and Social Security Disability Insurance (SSDI) alone cost the government almost $18 million for 4.1 million disabled recipients.[54] It has been estimated that pain is a factor in 40% to 60% of these claims by the time the cases reach closure (Social Security Administration [SSA], unpublished data).* This steady increase in volume of disability applications has been described as a "disability epidemic."[55]

SSA regulations define disability as an "inability to engage in any substantial gainful activity by reason of any medically determinable physical or mental impairment which can be expected to result in death or which has lasted or can be expected to last for a continuous period of not less than 12 months."[56] Therefore, impairments must be medically determinable, as established on the basis of medical or physical evidence. Medical evidence is defined as symptoms, signs, and laboratory findings,[57] but there must be medical signs or laboratory findings to establish that there is a medically determinable impairment. Even though an individual's symptoms are considered medical evidence, symptoms without corroborative medical signs or laboratory findings are currently insufficient to establish that there is a medically determinable impairment.[58]

SSA's pain policy, established in 1980, holds that pain is a symptom, not an impairment. In the absence of confirmatory medical signs or laboratory findings, chronic pain itself is not sufficient to demonstrate a physical or mental impairment. To be awarded disability benefits, the applicant must demonstrate a medically determinable impairment that could reasonably be expected to produce the alleged pain. Once a medically determinable impairment that could produce the pain is established, the limitations and restrictions due to pain must be considered.

Pain is a subjective phenomenon with a lack of reliable measures. Ambiguities in assessment strategies and variation in examinations used to identify physical or mental impairments have led to an increasing number of class action cases in the determination of disability involving the presence of pain (e.g., Moothart v Bowen[23] and Carr v Sullivan[59]). Variable judicial rulings led to congressional concern that a

---

*Unpublished data throughout this article refer to the final research reports to the funding agency—SSA, 1994.

standard for assessing the role of pain in the disability determination process would be established judicially rather than administratively on the basis of sound scientific and medical information. This concern precipitated §3 of Public Law 98-460,[25] which put into the statute SSA's long-standing pain policy. However, it additionally called for the appointment of a Commission on the Evaluation of Pain to work in consultation with the National Academy of Sciences Institute of Medicine (IOM) to evaluate the policy for evaluation of pain and recommend appropriate changes. The Pain Commission considered whether there should be a "listing" for impairment due primarily to pain within SSA's criteria for disability. The Pain Commission found that the SSA's policy was adequate and appropriate given the knowledge about pain, the absence of a reliable method to measure pain, and the fact that SSA did not have a uniform method to document pain.[5] The Pain Commission also observed the general lack of knowledge and understanding of chronic pain and pain behavior, the absence of a comprehensive database of chronic pain claimants, and inadequate SSA tools and techniques for obtaining information about pain. One of the primary recommendations was for SSA to conduct an experiment to develop the tools to remedy these deficiencies.

The Pain Commission recommended that the early stages of the determination process be redesigned to obtain more comprehensive information about pain and pain behavior by redesigning forms to alert interviewers and adjudicators to cases in which pain is a substantial element. They suggested the development of questionnaires to collect more information about pain at the earliest opportunity. They also recommended creation of a database on chronic pain patients to expand the knowledge of the phenomenon. They noted that because legal statutes and regulations are standard across the nation, the assessments and data collection should be equally standard and consistent.

The IOM recommended that a way be identified to factor subjective elements into the determination process in a more reliable and valid manner.[2] The Pain Commission also recommended general subjective criteria for the definition of impairment due primarily to pain.[5] These criteria included both elements that indicate evidence of pain as well as four categories of functional measures. Although these general criteria cannot be validated or tested for reliability, specific interpretations may be tested. These general criteria were embedded within the measurements of the present study, allowing for a validation of the recommendations.

Fishbain and colleagues[43] have effectively identified many of the methodological and logistical challenges inherent in efforts to predict the likelihood of return to work among individuals treated through Multidisciplinary Pain Centers. Definition problems such as difficulties in subcategorizing work outcome criteria to reflect full- and part-time work, vocational training, change in functional job status, as well as movement in and out of the work force, complicate efforts to isolate variables predictive of return to work. Variation in follow-up time intervals and the percentage of respondents participating in follow-up activities limit the ability to compare the effectiveness of various treatments. After reviewing 79 studies addressing work as a major outcome variable, the authors generated multiple recommendations designed to add methodological consistency and allow comparisons across various research protocols.

PAIN ASSESSMENT PROCESS

The ability to distinguish between individuals who are able or unable to work with chronic pain presents a unique challenge to the disability determination process. Because pain itself is subjective and is not directly measurable, prior assessment efforts have focused on a wide range of standard diagnostic and etiologic measures, patient self-reports, physician rating scales, and psychological measures. The many goals associated with the assessment and measurement of chronic pain are reflected in the variety of directions pain assessment research, and the development of pain assessment tools, has taken in recent years. Although a large number of different instruments have been used in pain research, two primary multidimensional pain assessment tools provided the foundation for chronic pain research in the 1980s. They are the McGill Pain Questionnaire (MPQ)[28] and the Multidimensional Pain Inventory (MPI).[29]

The MPQ is a patient self-report tool that elicits three types of measures of pain including: (a) the Pain Rating Index (PRI) based on the rank values of the words (pain adjectives) that add up to a score for each category, (b) the number of words actually chosen by the patient, and (c) the word combination chosen as the indicator of overall pain intensity at the time of administration of the questionnaire.[28] These measures are used to represent a quantitative index of pain.[28] Variable reliability has been reported for the MPQ and its subscales.[28,60,61] Multiple factor analyses have isolated five to seven subscales.[62–64]

The MPI is another patient self-assessment that combines multiple dimensions of assessment.[60,65,66] The MPI is divided into three parts with 13 empirically derived scales that address ratings of pain intensity, functional activities, affective distress, and several other dimensions. Part I contains five scales: reports of pain severity (PS scale), perceptions of how pain interferes with life (I scale), appraisals of the amount of support received from significant others (S scale), perceived life control (LC scale), and affective distress (AD scale). Part II contains the frequency of a range of behavioral responses by significant others to the patient's display of pain. Part III is an activities checklist that contains 19 common activities (GA scale). The MPI was designed to establish profiles of pain groups using the classification system of dysfunctional, interpersonally distressed, and adaptive coper.[29] The pain classification system employed in the MPI has been shown by Turk and Rudy,[29] as well as subsequent researchers,[67] to have good reliability and external validity.

Two instruments have received widespread use to assess patients with chronic pain from the physician's perspective. The Oswestry, Shropshire Low Back and Leg Pain Inventory[15] and the Summary of Nonorganic Physical Signs in Low Back Pain, also known as the Waddell,[39] are used primarily to measure low back pain. The 10-question Oswestry is designed to be completed by the examining physician who assesses the effects of low back and leg pain on daily living. The utility of the Oswestry has been documented by its widespread clinical use.[15,68,69] The Waddell, also completed by the examining physician, is a standardized group of five types of nonorganic signs (tenderness, simulation, distraction, regional, and overreaction) that patients with low back pain may display. A finding of three or more signs is clinically significant. Waddell initially validated this instrument through four studies conducted in Canada, Scotland, and Great Britain.[68]

Attention has shifted in recent years to the psychological component of chronic pain assessment, as opposed to the direct diagnosis and etiology measurement for patients with acute pain.[35] Quite frequently both pain researchers and pain treatment centers administer a brief psychological or social assessment in addition to the instruments that are specifically related to pain. Although a multitude of instruments are available, this study used the Center for Epidemiological Studies Depression Scale (CES-D)[34] and the Family Adaptability & Cohesion Evaluation Scale (FACES III),[70] both of which have been extensively validated[70,71] and are known to be reliable.[72,73]

The use of one or more of the aforementioned instruments, coupled with the clinical impressions of examining physicians, assists in the assessment of individuals with chronic pain. However, as Fishbain and colleagues[43] have noted, there remains a vital need for a standardized and multidimensional assessment battery that addresses the previously mentioned methodological challenges and more accurately predicts the ability of individuals to perform substantial gainful activity. Present research studies and treatment programs use multiple measures to fully assess the domains encompassed by the study or program. This unfortunately leads to an increased volume of paperwork because some assessments overlap for some domains and decrease comparability of outcomes across studies and between programs. Variability of outcome measured also makes comparison difficult.

The Multiperspective Multidimensional Pain Assessment Protocol (MMPAP) (KS Rucker et al., unpublished data, 1994) is a recently developed assessment tool that builds on previous evaluation efforts.

The MMPAP is unique in that it collects and uses information from a variety of sources yet retains the distinctive multidimensional quality that is so effective as a component of the MPI and MPQ. Patient self-report, physician ratings of patient behavior, results of a standardized medical examination, and physician clinical appraisal of rehabilitation potential are all combined in an attempt to obtain information from a variety of perspectives.

Major domains assessed in the protocol include rating of pain dimensions, medical information, mental health status, social support networks, functional limitations and abilities, and rehabilitation potential. Extensive validation analyses have been completed on the MMPAP, and the protocol has demonstrated high reliability, construct validity, and concurrent validity (KS Rucker et al., unpublished data, 1994).[74–76] These initial validation and reliability results will be reviewed briefly.

The MMPAP has been standardized and tested for reliability and validity. The purpose of this article is to report the predictive ability of the MMPAP to identify those disability applicants with chronic pain who will return to work and to identify the items within the MMPAP that most accurately predict future employment outcomes. The standardized MMPAP was used to assess the chronic pain dimensions of 599 nationally selected SSA disability applicants who claimed pain related to the impairment for which they were applying for disability compensation and to predict the employment outcomes of those applicants 6 months after disability decision.

METHODS

Sample

The MMPAP was administered to a total of 691 SSA disability applicants from across the nation. All participants had chronic pain, strictly defined within this study to be pain of a duration of 6 months or greater, regardless of initial cause of the pain. Because the study centered on employment or return to work, all participants were adults of working age who had not taken early retirement. Working age was defined as 18 to 64 years of age.

The high prevalence of chronic low back complaints has prompted many researchers to concentrate on this specific problem. A recent meta-analysis of published outcome studies from multidisciplinary pain treatment centers reviewed 65 independent studies that primarily emphasized chronic back pain.[77] However, disability applicants who claim pain experience a wide range of pain intensities and locations, the most difficult claims to resolve being those that involve pain inconsistent with the medical evidence.[78] It was therefore imperative that the present research address the full spectrum of pain complaints, including those with unknown etiology. To allow for a variety of pain complaints and simultaneously maintain a manageable sample size, although patients were randomly solicited, every other patient who applied for disability in the sample pool with a low back pain complaint was selected for participation. This selection constraint allowed the complex statistical analyses to be performed on a wide spectrum of chronic pain conditions without the need for a prohibitively large sample size.[79]

The sample was stratified to be representative of SSA's claimant population for the demographic variables of gender, age, and ethnic origin. Prior research on both the prevalence of chronic pain and the likelihood of return to work[80,81] has indicated a significant correlation with advancing age. Additionally, this study was designed to identify predictors of return to work without regard to cultural, ethnic, or gender bias. Therefore, the sample was stratified to be representative of the SSA disability applicant population for these demographics.

The sample was divided equally between SSDI applicants and SSI or concurrent (both SSDI and SSI) applicants. Because SSI applicants are not required to have worked previously, whereas SSDI applicants must have a history of prior work to receive disability benefits, it was important that the sample represent both groups. All claimants within the study were identified as initial applicants for disability benefits. Follow-up interviews were completed with 603 (87% of the sample) applicants a minimum of 6 months after disability decision (average follow-up time span was 8 months). Table 6-1 summarizes key demographic information for the final sample.

To maintain external validity, the MMPAP was tested at six national sites. The sites were chosen to obtain a representative cross section of disability applicants. One site was chosen in each of 6 of the 10 SSA regions, and the chosen sites reflected the variation (centralized versus decentralized disability determination offices) in the SSA disability determination process. The site locations were Indianapolis, Indiana; St. Louis, Missouri; Albuquerque, New Mexico; Philadelphia, Pennsylvania; Richmond, Virginia; and Seattle, Washington.

Instrumentation
A multiphase process was used to develop, standardize, and validate the MMPAP. The questionnaires for this study originated with the Pain Commission's suggestions for items or indicators that were hypothesized as potentially helpful in pain assessment. This initial list of items was then expanded by a national team of pain experts in a series of roundtable discussions to create a comprehensive list. After a pilot study in which the protocol was administered to 67 chronic pain patients,[82] the protocol was revised to improve clarity and reduce ambiguity and redundancy. The revised protocol was subsequently administered to a total of 651 outpatients with chronic pain recruited

Table 6-1   Demographic Composition of the Postdecision Subsample (n = 603)

Demographic Description	Frequency	Percentage
Ethnic origin		
American Indian	15	2.5
Asian	3	0.5
Black	183	30.3
Hispanic	60	10.0
White	336	55.7
Other	6	1.0
Sex		
Male	318	52.7
Female	285	47.3
Age (y)		
<40	213	35.3
40–54	250	41.5
≥55	140	23.2
Employment status at assessment		
Employed	36	6.0
Unemployed	567	94.0

from clinics at a major medical institution. All participants were adults of working age, 18 to 64 years old. To assess the related elements of those individuals who remain employed although they have pain, as well as those who are not employed, the sample was a priori selected as half employed and half not employed.

Reliability
Rater reliability was tested to ensure that the MMPAP and methods provided consistent information. Twenty percent of the participating patients were randomly selected for a second recruitment to once again undergo the battery of assessments for reliability analyses. The reliability patients were chosen randomly and were demographically similar to the entire sample. The second assessment was completed an average of 31 days after the first. Reliability analyses revealed that the assessments were measuring stable constructs, as indicated by the similarity of responses with repeated assessments, both with the same administrator and physicians and with different administrators and physicians.[74] The statistics used were the Cohen's κ and the weighted Cohen's κ (for variables with continuously scaled response options) rater reliability.[81]

Construct Validity

To assess the construct validity of the MMPAP principal factor analysis[84] with varimax, rotation of factors was performed on the protocol responses.[75] Because it was anticipated that the patients' responses would be correlated with the physicians' responses, two independent analyses were performed. The resulting factors within an analysis were uncorrelated. Kaiser's MSA,[85] which was computed before analysis, confirmed the adequacy of sample size for all analyses with a value of 0.93 for the patient's perspective and a value of 0.89 from the physician's perspective.

Twelve factors were retained by the factor analysis of the patient's perspective, with eigen values ranging from 5.81 to 1.17. In decreasing order of factor strength, the factors were related to pain descriptions, functional abilities, effects on activities of daily living (ADL), environmental components, mood alteration, emotional descriptors, family history, significant other actions, effect on cognitive processes, functional repetitions, significant other reactions, and pain interference with sleep. Eight factors were retained by the factor analysis of the physicians' perspective, eigen values ranging from 4.68 to 1.17. The factors were related to perception of functional abilities/restrictions, motivation causes and effects, effects on emotional status/cognitive processes, treatment modalities, musculoskeletal indicators, autonomic and vascular indicators, pain descriptors, and tenderness and spasms.

The majority of items remained components of their originally conceptualized domains. As a result of the factor analyses, the functional limitations domain was subsequently divided into two domains: (a) functional limitations and ADL, including an assessment of the effect of pain on the patient's concentration and cognitive processes, ADL, and emotional status as it relates to function, primarily as perceived by the patient; and (b) functional abilities, which assess functional abilities of the patient as perceived primarily by the physicians.

Concurrent Validity

Because there is currently no single comprehensive pain measurement instrument available that spans the breadth of the present protocol, it was necessary to use several standardized instruments that focus on specific aspects of the pain experience to assess concurrent validity of related domains in the MMPAP.[76] The instruments used were the MPQ, the MPI, the CES-D, the FACES III, the Oswestry, and the Waddell (KS Rucker et al., unpublished data, 1994). Concurrent validity was obtained with a target rate of 0.70 Pearson's correlation coefficient between all relevant domains on each of the aforementioned instruments, and the equivalent domains of the MMPAP (KS Rucker et al., unpublished data, 1994).[76]

Content Validity

The final analysis performed on this initial set of pain patients was a preliminary content validity analysis. A follow-up interview was performed 6 months after assessment, primarily to ascertain the patient's status with respect to the three outcome variables: whether the patient was employed, whether the patient's employment status had changed, and whether the patient's pain level had changed. A discriminant function analysis was then performed to determine which assessment variables were most predictive of these three outcome variables. Results of the validity phase content validity analysis revealed 120 highly predictive variables. These were later tested on the national SSA claimant sample. Because it was anticipated that a much larger percentage of claimants will remain unemployed 6 months after disability decision, the results of these early content validity analyses, in which 50% of the sample was employed with pain at assessment, were used to create the variable list analyzed in the national validity phase. With this additional step, variables were included in the final prediction equation that predict possible employment although chronic pain persists.[86]

Criterion Variables

The criterion measures used for this study were two employment-based indicators and one pain-level indicator. SSA claimants were recruited as soon as possible after disability application and were recontacted a minimum of 6 months after a decision was received from SSA to determine the outcome of each criterion measure. Employment status, designated as employed or not employed, and change in employment status, which takes into consideration movement from part-time to full-time status, both were assessed. Although all participants had chronic pain, pain intensity varied. Change in that intensity in terms of better, same, and worse was examined as the third criterion.

Domains

The structure of the MMPAP consists of individual items combined into domains. The initial items and domains were based on expert panel recommendations and literature review, and were subsequently slightly modified by factor analysis,[75] the results of which are briefly described in the previous section. Each of these domains is briefly described in the following paragraphs.

The rating of pain dimensions domain includes pain description items such as frequency, length, intensity and unpleasantness, psychological perception of pain, pain behaviors, perception of control over pain, and pain interference with sleep. This information is collected through both patient reports and physician ratings. The mental health status domain includes the patient's self-report of depressive symptoms, contact with the mental health system, substance abuse, and sociopathy. This domain also includes the physicians' perception of patient depression, substance abuse, and other mental health indicators. The social support networks domain includes the patient's perception of support provided by his or her significant other, the patient's perception of the significant other's reaction to the patient, and each physician's perception of the patient's social support network.

The medical information domain is primarily a series of questions related to the physical examination that each physician performs. It also includes health care use, use of medication, and willingness to tolerate painful medical procedures as collected through patient reports and physician ratings, diagnostic testing, and cause of pain. The functional limitations domain includes an assessment of the effect of pain on the patient's concentration and cognitive processes, ADL, and emotional status perceived by the patient and physicians. The functional abilities domain contains primarily functional abilities and ADL as perceived by the patient and physicians. The employment or rehabilitation potential domain contains the perceptions of the physicians regarding the patient's employment potential and motivation to work. This was assessed with several questions regarding the patient's effort level, whether the patient has obtained maximum medical improvement or would do so in the next 6 months, and the patient's work-related functional level.

Procedure: National Study Plan

Sample

The SSA provided weekly lists of applicants for disability benefits within the six target regions. The lists were screened to identify applicants of working age with chronic pain related to the condition for which they were applying for disability, with available transportation or a residence within a 1-hour radius of the test site. Claimants with the necessary criteria for the study were entered into a data pool.

The SSA continued to provide weekly data for as long as was necessary to maintain a sufficiently ample pool of applicants. Approximately 25% of the pool were then selected through a stratified random process to participate in the study. The sample was stratified by national SSA demographics for age, race, and gender. The percentage selected from each site was proportional to the SSA service area for that site.

Those claimants selected were informed of the study and were offered $50 to attend one of our research clinics to receive two separate physician examinations and to complete the additional data forms. Thirty-five percent (489) of the 1400 applicants approached refused participation. An additional 14% consented to participate but later declined participation; included in this percentage are two claimants who had died since agreeing to participate. A total of 710 individuals participated, for a response rate of 51%. However, the data for 19 subjects were eliminated before analysis because the subjects were inappropriate for the study (e.g., the pain was due to cancer, the subject had taken early retirement, the subject did not have chronic pain), for a final sample size of 691. Decision information was obtained for all 1400 applicants. There was not a significant difference in award rate between respondents and nonrespondents.

Data Collection
Data were collected from a variety of perspectives. The patient supplied basic demographic and vocational information on a referral form and completed an additional patient instrument containing pain information, both historically and at the time of assessment. Two physician instruments were completed, one representing information that could be obtained from the individual's treating physician (e.g., willingness to undergo painful and invasive interventions) and one representing information that would be provided by a consulting physician during the disability application process.

The patient provided an assessment of history, location, frequency, duration, severity, and intensity of pain with exacerbating factors; history of health care use for diagnosis and treatment of pain (i.e., surgical, pharmaceutical, physician visits, hospitalizations); current usage and future need for health care use; pain behaviors before and since onset of pain; cognitive status and ability for task completion; emotional disturbance before and since the onset of pain; history of mental health intervention; ADL and social functioning before and since the onset of pain; and functional ability and limitations.

Each physician completed a full physical examination after a standardized protocol and then completed a questionnaire and examination form that included the evaluation of the following patient characteristics: pain complaint, including sensory and affective intensity; frequency and duration of pain; use of health care systems; exhibition of pain behaviors; emotional status; cognitive and functional status; ability to complete a task; physical examination and evidence of physical impairment; laboratory and imaging data supporting patient's pain complaint; and functional ability and rehabilitation potential. The treating physician also completed a historical section that outlined previous services, treatments, and medications.

Follow-up interviews were conducted by telephone or mail. The target follow-up time was 6 months after the claimant's decision date for disability benefits. Information about the disability decision (i.e., award or denial, date of decision, and disability code) was obtained from the SSA national database. The claimant was primarily asked about pain intensity and unpleasantness, employment and litigation statuses, and efforts to gain employment since the initial assessment.

Predictive Validity Analyses

A discriminant function analysis was performed with the items that compose each of the individual instruments as predictor variables. The discriminant function, also referred to as a classification criterion, is created by generating a measure of generalized squared distance, which creates approximately multivariate normal distributions. Three primary outcomes 6 months after decision were tested. The specific outcomes or criterion variables addressed were: (a) whether the claimant was employed; (b) whether the claimant's employment situation was the same or better than at assessment; and (c) whether the claimant's pain intensity was the same, better, or worse than at assessment.

RESULTS

Subsample Identified at Follow-up

The average follow-up time was 8 months after disability decision. At the conclusion of follow-up data collection, 10 claimants were excluded from the final analyses. Two individuals had not received a decision, four had received the decision less than 6 months before the end of the project, and four were deceased at follow-up. Additionally, a total of 78 claimants were lost to follow-up either because they refused to answer follow-up questions or because they could not be located. Comparisons of this reduced sample with the original sample indicated no demographic deviations. Although the entire postdecision follow-up sample size was 603, four individuals had excessive missing information on the original assessment or the follow-up questionnaire, reducing the effective sample size of these analyses to 599.

The percentage of claimants in this sample who were awarded disability was 22.8 (157), with 77.2% (532) being denied disability. Two claimants had not received a decision at the culmination of follow-up data collection. There had been concern expressed that individuals awarded benefits would be disproportionately followed because they would be less likely to move without a forwarding address. However, χ^2 analyses showed no significance between those contacted at follow-up in terms of the disposition of their claims (i.e., between the subgroup denied benefits and those approved for benefits).

The ratio of denials to allowances was equivalent to SSA decision statistics at approximately three to one (Table 6-2). Table 6-2 also compares criterion variable change status between awards and denials. The pain level changes did not vary with disability award, and as expected a higher percentage of those denied disability were employed 6 months postdecision. Also as anticipated, a much larger percentage of claimants remained unemployed 6 months after disability decision than were employed. This anticipated result was prepared for in two ways. First, the results of the early content validity

Table 6-2   Criterion Variable Status by Social Security Administration Decision Results

Criterion Variable	Allowed (n = 140)		Denied (n = 459)	
	n	%	n	%
Pain level change				
Better	32	22.9	90	19.6
Same	64	45.7	191	39.4
Worse	44	31.4	188	41.0
Employment status				
Employed	9	6.4	66	14.4
Not employed	131	93.6	393	85.6
Employment change				
Better	7	5.0	52	11.3
Same	129	92.1	396	86.3

analyses from the early validity phase, in which 50% of the sample was employed with pain at assessment, was used to create the variable list analyzed in the national validity phase. This preparatory analysis allowed for the inclusion of predictive variables that indicated the individuals who were able to work, even though chronic pain persisted. Second, in running the statistical analysis for the national validity phase, it was not assumed that half of the claimants would be employed and half would be unemployed at follow-up. The actual percentages of each category were used in the prediction of who would fall into each category.

Predictive Validity

The discriminant ability of the final set of predictors was considerably greater than chance for all three criterion variables when the outcomes of the same set of claimants were predicted 6 months after decision. Table 6-3 displays the predictive validity distribution for the criterion variables.

The results indicated that there were approximately 60 to 65 variables that contributed significantly to the outcome prediction of each of the three criterion variables, a total of 116 variables predicting the outcome of one or more of the criterion variables. Table 6-4 sorts the variables into 65 items by classifying the variables within the table by source. Each physician's assessment is considered a separate variable, independent from the claimant's response.

It was theorized that if this set of instruments actually predicts the criterion variables, the outcomes of those who are denied disability will be predicted more accurately than outcomes of those who are

Table 6-3 Predictive Ability of Multiperspective Multidimensional Pain Assessment Protocol for Each Criterion Variable Outcome

Criterion Variable	Discriminant Ability (%)
Employed or unemployed?	
Employed	36.0
Unemployed	97.9
Overall	90.2
Has employment situation changed?	
Better	44.1
Same	98.3
Overall	92.8
Has pain intensity changed?	
Better	51.6
Same	67.8
Worse	67.7
Overall	64.4

awarded disability, because there will be the additional disincentive of the disability award. This is balanced by the smaller sample of those awarded disability when using the same sample to predict.

DISCUSSION

Chronic pain has always presented a challenge to physicians from the standpoint of definition, classification, diagnosis, and treatment. The responsibility of physicians to determine permanent impairment and to provide recommendations regarding the likelihood of returning to work is made more difficult by the complexities presented by the chronic pain patient. For physicians to address these needs, information must be obtained from a variety of areas including mental health status, coping mechanisms, social supports network, functional limitations and abilities, rehabilitation potential, and other factors.

The assessment protocol described in this study was developed and validated under contract from SSA and was designed to address the concerns raised in the reports by the Commission on Evaluation of Pain and the Institute of Medicine Committee Report on Pain and Disability. The purpose of the present study was to apply the MMPAP to a population of disability applicants to determine the extent to which the protocol could be routinely and uniformly used to predict the likelihood that a disability applicant with chronic pain would return to work. Discriminant validity analyses indicate a high level of discriminative power within the assessment protocol with respect to employment status and

Table 6-4 Predictive Value of Each Protocol Question

Description of Question	Who Answers	Predictive Value
Rating of pain dimensions		
Frequency of pain (past 6 months)	C, P	E, S
Length of pain-free periods (past 6 months)	C	E, S
How long pain lasts (past 6 months)	C	I
Unpleasantness during usual pain intensity (past week)	C	S
Unpleasantness during highest pain intensity (past week)	C	E, I, S
Usual intensity of pain	C, P	
How often pain awakened patient (past 6 months)	C, P	S
Degree patient has talked about pain	C, P	E, I, S
Degree patient displays nervousness due to pain	P	I, S
Mental health status domain		
How often patient felt hopeless (past week)	C	E, S
How often patient felt he/she would never work again (past week)	C	E, S
How often patient felt he/she would never do enjoyed things	C	E, S
How often patient felt depressed (past 6 months)	C	E, S
How severely patient felt anxious (past 6 months)	C, P	S
How patient feels about self	C	E, I, S
How patient's appetite is now	C	E, S
Degree patient has exhibited mood alterations	P	E, I, S
Social support networks domain		
How often significant other gets irritated because of patient's pain	C	I, S
How often significant other gets frustrated because of patient's pain	C	I, S
Level of difficulty in relationship with spouse/ significant other due to pain	C, P	I, S
Medical examination findings domain		
Level of joint deformity	P	E, I, S
Level of gait abnormalities	P	E, I, S
Amount of support a computed tomographic scan gives to complaints	P	
Amount of support radiographs give to complaints	P	E, S
Amount of support electrodiagnosis gives to complaints	P	I, S

continues

Table 6-4   Predictive Value of Each Protocol Question *continued*

Description of Question	Who Answers	Predictive Value
Functional limitations—ADL domain		
How much climbing stairs causes pain	C	E, I, S
How much bending, stooping, kneeling cause pain	C	I, S
How much talking and listening cause pain	C	I
How pushing and pulling affect patient while in pain	C	I, S
How climbing stairs affects patient while in pain	C	S
How handling and feeling affect patient while in pain	C	E, S
How talking and listening affect patient while in pain	C	I
How often pain limited patient's concentration	C	E, I
How often pain limited patient's toleration of minor irritations	C	I
How often patient feels frustrated (past 6 months)	C	I
How often patient attended recreational activities (before pain)	C	I
How well patient can make decisions now	C	I
Level of difficulty in heavy household tasks due to pain	C, P	
Level of difficulty in moving about the house due to pain	C, P	I, S
Level of difficulty in traveling independently about town	C, P	S
Level of difficulty in interpersonal relationships due to pain	P	E, I
Level of difficulty in remembering instructions due to pain	C, P	S
Functional abilities domain		
Hours the patient can stand	P	E, I, S
Hours the patient can walk	P	I
Hours the patient can push	P	E, I, S
Hours the patient can pull	P	E, I, S
Hours the patient can stand and walk	P	E, S
Hours the patient can work overhead	P	I
Hours the patient can sit	P	E, I, S
Hours the patient can do simple grasping	P	E, I, S
Hours the patient can do fine hand manipulations	P	E, I, S

continues

Table 6-4   Predictive Value of Each Protocol Question *continued*

Description of Question	Who Answers	Predictive Value
Max. weight patient can lift floor to counter occasionally	P	E, I, S
Max. weight patient can lift floor to counter repetitively	P	E, I, S
Max. weight patient can lift counter to counter occasionally	P	S
Max. weight patient can lift counter to counter repetitively	P	E, I, S
Max. weight patient can lift counter to overhead occasionally	P	E, I
Max. weight patient can lift counter to overhead repetitively	P	E, I, S
Minutes patient can stand without a break	P	I, S
Minutes patient can sit without a break	P	E, S
Employment or rehabilitation potential domain		
Level of effort patient will expend for FCE	P	E, I, S
When maximum medical improvement can be expected	P	I
Pain complaints greater than from objective clinical findings	P	I
Level of treatment required in the next year	P	E, I, S
Level of treatment required in the future (indefinitely)	P	I
Pain behaviors appear exaggerated	P	I

ADL, activities of daily living; *C*, claimant answers the question; *P*, both physicians answer the question; *E*, the answer is predictive of whether the claimant will be employed or unemployed 6 months after disability decision; *S*, the answer is predictive of whether the claimant's employment situation will change; *I*, the answer is predictive of whether the claimant's pain intensity will change; *FCE*, functional capacity evaluation.

pain intensity approximately 8 months after disability award. Although no prediction can be 100% accurate on the individual applicant level, the protocol aids in the prediction of future employment and pain status by estimating the likelihood of each of the future status categories.

This study adds considerably to past research of this type partially because this study controlled for the demographic differences of age, gender, and race rather than using them in the prediction of the outcomes of the criterion variables. In this way, the predictive ability of items that can be addressed by a multidisciplinary pain team, such as psychological or ADL variables, can be measured. It was found that many of the psychological and ADL items are significant predictors, although they may have been masked by one of the demographic variables in prior studies or were not assessed in prior investigations.

The results of the predictive analyses illustrate the diversity and complexity of factors that contribute to the likelihood that a disability applicant will return to work or experience a change in the intensity of pain. Both patient and physician ratings of pain dimensions contributed significantly to an individual's postdecision employment status. Specifically, these predictive variables were frequency of pain and degree that the patient has talked about pain, as reported by both the patient and the physician, and the patient's assessment of length of pain-free periods and unpleasantness during highest pain intensity. Ratings of pain intensity and unpleasantness at the time of assessment did not contribute substantially to subsequent changes in an individual's pain intensity.

Medical information obtained from the standardized physician's examination revealed a number of items that contributed to the predictive power of the protocol. The physicians assessments of the level of joint deformity and level of gait abnormalities were related to the likelihood that the individual will obtain employment after decision.

The patient's assessment of his or her present psychological status had a dramatic effect on subsequent employment status. Individuals who expressed feelings of hopelessness, depression, and concerns that they would never work again were far less likely than other applicants to be working at follow-up. In contrast, these variables did not contribute to the prediction of changes in the individual's pain intensity. This finding provides empirical support for the importance of an individual's ability to cope with and adapt to his or her pain as a significant determinant of the level of disability that results from physical ailments.[2,35] The patient's assessment of social support network contributed little predictive power in any of the three discriminative analyses. Only the level of difficulty experienced by the individual in his or her relationship with spouse or significant other contributed to subsequent changes in pain intensity and employment status.

The patient's assessment of the extent to which his or her pain resulted in functional limitations in the ability to perform ADL had little impact on whether he or she was employed at follow-up. However, these items contributed significantly to an individual's reported change in pain intensity. Conversely, the physicians' ratings of functional abilities had high predictive ability for both employment status and change in pain intensity as well as change in employment status. These findings indicate the importance of obtaining both the patient's and the physicians' perspective to maximize the predictive power of a pain assessment protocol.

Finally, the physicians' subjective, clinical appraisal of employment or rehabilitation potential also contributed to the results of the content validity analysis. Physicians' perceptions of the level of treatment required by the patient in the coming year and the degree to which pain complaints were exaggerated or were greater than might be expected from clinical findings contributed to the prediction of changes in pain intensity. Both level of treatment required in the next year and anticipated level of effort a patient would expend in a functional capacity evaluation significantly contributed to the ability to predict employment at follow-up. If an increase in the level of treatment in the next year is anticipated, the patient is less likely to be employed at follow-up. Those individuals who were predicted to go beyond maximum effort and expend extreme effort during functional capacity examinations are less likely to be employed at follow-up.

Limitations of the Study

The sample of the present study comprised only individuals who had applied for disability benefits. As such, the results of the study should not be generalized to all chronic pain patients. The sample was stratified to ensure that it was representative of SSA disability applicants on key demographic variables such as age, gender, and ethnicity. To allow the generalization to the entirety of the SSA applicant population, the number of individuals with low back pain in the sample was controlled.

The study did not control for medical or other interventions (vocational or psychological) during the period between the initial assessment and the follow-up interview. The study was designed as a nonintervention subjective analysis, and any attempts to deny individual treatment regimens as a control would have been cost-prohibitive as well as inhumane. This design reflects existing circumstances of the SSA disability determination offices when working with claimants who allege pain.

The conclusion that the physicians' ratings of functional abilities had high predictive ability may be viewed with skepticism by some clinicians. It must be emphasized that all physicians within this study had physical medicine and rehabilitation training, as well as training specific to this study. The questions were not asked in isolation but rather were a component of a series of topical questions as well as a physical examination. Individual questions should not be interpreted outside of this context. These findings also indicate the importance of obtaining both the patients' and physicians' perspectives to maximize the predictive power of a pain assessment protocol.

Implications of the Study

The study has practical implications for the disability determination process, as well as for the treatment of individuals with chronic pain. The results of the content validation analysis indicated that the MMPAP is a valid clinical tool when administered by physicians trained in the use of the protocol. Some experience with chronic pain, disability issues, and functional assessment is preferable for the physicians. To ensure reliability in administration, the physicians and support staff were provided an intensive, 8-hour training session before using the forms. Clinical utility is enhanced by the fact that the MMPAP does not involve expensive or high-technology equipment but is simply a structured, multidimensional examination and questionnaire.

Use of this protocol with chronic pain patients should give the clinician the ability to accurately and consistently assess likelihood of returning to work early in the medical evaluation. This may have an impact on the choices of treatment plans. For example, patients who were identified as not likely to return to work could receive psychological, vocational, comprehensive rehabilitation or behavioral interventions earlier than they would otherwise. The hope is that use of appropriate clinical interventions earlier in the process will improve clinical outcome and return-to-work rates.

The protocol could assist in studies to assess whether various rehabilitation interventions are effective. Identification of patients as unlikely to return to work by a valid and reliable instrument could assist in finding interventions that subsequently change the outcome predicted.[47] A baseline assessment and prediction would be obtained with the protocol, identifying those individuals with a poor prognosis, who would therefore most likely benefit from interventions. Subsequent to the intervention or treatment, the protocol would again be administered and compared with the baseline assessment, to determine whether the predicted outcome had indeed changed. Use of the MMPAP in medical rehabilitation research to assist in proving the value of various treatments would be very beneficial. This is especially true now that third-party payers are demanding increased evidence of the effectiveness of expensive interventions.

The existing SSA disability determination process has often resulted in benefits' eventually being awarded to chronic pain claimants through the courts. Benefits were awarded, usually several years after initial application, when the administrative law judge had the advantage of seeing that the claimant had not returned to work in the interim. The process delays awarding benefits to claimants who allege pain and create additional costs for SSA. The use of a standardized pain assessment protocol such as the MMPAP early in the disability determination process would reduce the number of time-consuming and expensive appeals and readjudications. Pain would be comprehensively considered consistently and fairly for all applications. Perhaps more importantly, subsequent research may enable SSA to identify claimants with chronic pain who would benefit from vocational, psychological, behavioral, or other interventions.

CONCLUSION

A major need identified by the Commission or Evaluation of Pain, the Institute of Medicine, and the SSA has been a valid, reliable, multidimensional assessment tool that predicts return to work in the chronic pain patient. It is apparent that there is a great need for a rational and consistent decision-making process in the area of chronic pain and disability. Inconsistencies exist in physical examinations performed, history-taking techniques, and interpretation of examination and history findings for chronic pain. It is not surprising that there is wide variation in impairment ratings and disability assessments. In this time of limited resources and of increasing needs, decisions regarding resources for chronic pain patients (disability benefits, pain treatment centers, etc.) must be made and are being made on a daily basis.

This study has shown that in the performance of a standardized protocol physician evaluation, input is crucial in predicting likelihood of return to work. Doctors are being asked to provide information and recommendations for workers compensation carriers, federal agencies, and the judiciary system without regard to standardized assessment. These groups have varying levels of training, knowledge, and experience about pain and disability. Consistent or rational data collection to support or guide the decisions has not existed. These decisions ultimately have an impact on the psychosocial, physical, and economic aspects of patients' lives as well as on the economics of business, industry, and government. Future research is needed to confirm and extend the results of the present investigation in a way that will improve the responsiveness of the SSA disability determination process for individuals with chronic pain.

Standardization of Chronic Pain Assessment: A Multiperspective Approach

Karen S. Rucker, M.D., Helen M. Metzler, M.S., and John Kregel, Ed.D.*

This article is reprinted for the purposes of providing manual users with resources regarding validity of PAI. The MMPAP in this chapter is referred to as the PAI elsewhere in this manual.

ABSTRACT

Objective
This study reports the results of reliability and validity analyses on the Multiperspective Multidimensional Pain Assessment Protocol (MMPAP). When pain becomes chronic, it intertwines with the many dimensions of a patient's life, increasing the complexity of the patient's perception of the pain and, subsequently, the prescribed treatment. Both the patient's perspective and the physician's perspective are crucial in the assessment of these multiple dimensions, creating a fundamental need for a valid and reliable, multiperspective, multidimensional pain assessment tool.

*Reprinted with permission from KS Rucker, HM Metzler, and J Kregel. Standardization of chronic pain assessment: A multiperspective approach. *Clin J Pain* 1996;12: 94–110.

From the Department of Physical Medicine and Rehabilitation and Rehabilitation Research and Training Center, Virginia Commonwealth University/Medical College of Virginia, Richmond, Virginia.

Manuscript submitted October 13, 1994; 1st revision received April 20, 1995; 2nd revision received March 19, 1996; accepted for publication March 21, 1996.

This work was sponsored by the Social Security Administration under Contract 600-90-0229. Additional support was provided by the National Institutes of Health General Clinical Research Centers at Virginia Commonwealth University/Medical College of Virginia (VCU/MCV) under NCRR grant MO I RR 00065.

Design

A randomized regional sample of outpatients complaining of chronic pain. Each MMPAP consisted of physical examinations by two physicians and the participant's subjective self-report. Primary criterion standards were the Multidimensional Pain Instrument and the McGill Pain Questionnaire.

Setting

Ambulatory referral centers, both public and private.

Participants

A population-based random sample of 651 outpatients claiming chronic pain. Thirty-six patients who were originally recruited refused participation, and four patients did not complete the entire assessment.

Interventions

No interventions were continued or initiated by the research team.

Main Outcome Measures

Because this was a validation of the instruments used, no patient outcomes were influenced or assessed. The MMPAP is a recently developed pain assessment protocol that uses both subjective information and objective medical evidence.

Results

The MMPAP proved to be a reliable and valid tool that may assist in the assessment of chronic pain when two physicians independently assess the patient and this information is combined with the patient's self-reported pain perceptions. Test-retest and interrater reliability analyses confirmed that the data collected with the MMPAP were repeatable. A combination of concurrent comparisons with previously validated instruments, construct corroboration with factor analysis, and internal consistency analyses ascertained the validity of the MMPAP.

Conclusions

The introduction of this standardized protocol will assist in standardizing assessments of patients with chronic pain. The MMPAP has potential as a diagnostic tool, a measure of treatment effectiveness, and a tool to compare various pain treatment center outcomes.

Key Words

Chronic pain, reliability, standardized assessment, validation.

INTRODUCTION

The inability to meet adult role expectations because of chronic pain represents a large and growing problem. Functional limitations due to pain disrupt the lives of thousands of individuals each year and challenge the nation's health care system. In a recent poll of Americans concerning their experience with severe pain, nearly one quarter of adults said that they experience pain strong enough to interfere with their daily activities every month.[52] Eighty-three percent of people reporting persistent pain reported that they had pain longer than a year.[2] For individuals with pain who have jobs, it has been estimated that pain causes more than $55 billion a year in lost workdays.[3]

Accurate assessment of chronic pain is critical for a variety of reasons and may take many forms. The many goals associated with the assessment and measurement of chronic pain are reflected in the variety of directions pain assessment research and the development of pain assessment tools have taken in recent years. First, as with acute pain, chronic pain assessment is a diagnostic tool.[4,8,9] Individual clinicians use short questionnaires, checklists, or other devices to obtain relevant diagnostic information on individual patients, many of which they have developed themselves[10,11] or which they have modified or compiled based on existing instruments.[12] Second, treatment effectiveness is often measured by changes in pain or reported pain levels. Brief but easily repeatable assessment tools such as the visual analogue scale,[13] the Functional Independence Measure,[14] and the Oswestry[15] have been used to document the effectiveness of various treatment protocols. Finally, an accurate pain assessment tool may be used to assess function[16] and predict functional abilities[17] and related consequential actions, such as disability assessment,[18,19] workers compensation, formalized pain research,[20,21] and pain treatment center evaluation.[22]

Ambiguities in assessment strategies and variation in examinations used to identify physical or mental impairments have led to increased litigation related to the determination of disability involving the presence of pain.[23,24] Variable judicial rulings led to congressional concern that a standard for assessing the role of pain in the disability determination process would be established judicially, rather than administratively, based on sound scientific and medical information. This concern precipitated section 3 of Public Law 98-460,[25] which put into statutes the long-standing pain policy of the Social Security Administration (SSA) but called for the appointment of a Commission on the Evaluation of Pain[5] to work in consultation with the National Academy of Sciences Institute of Medicine[2] to evaluate the policy for evaluation of pain and recommend appropriate changes.

Chronic pain and its definition are problematical due to a lack of consensus about basic definitions and inconsistencies in measurement and assessment techniques. Although considerable effort has been put into a taxonomy to help classify various pain symptoms,[26,27] at present no classification system for chronic pain, musculoskeletal disorders, or the most common subgroup of chronic pain, back pain, is uniformly used. Since pain is subjective and is not directly measurable, prior assessment efforts have focused on a wide range of standard diagnostic and etiologic indicators, patient self-reports, physician rating scales, and psychological assessment tools. With few exceptions,[28–30] most diagnostic tools and assessment forms for chronic pain assess a single domain related to the pain. Many instruments are used as a subjective assessment of pain dimensions, including frequency, duration, intensity and unpleasantness, psychological perception of pain, pain behaviors, perception of control over pain, and pain interference with sleep.[31–33] Other instruments specifically assess mental health status, such as the patient's self-report of depressive symptoms, contact with the mental health system, substance abuse, and sociopathy.[34–36] Some instruments address the patient's social support network, including support provided by the patient's significant other and the significant other's reaction to the patient.[37] Diagnostic protocols used to record medical information related to the physical examination may also include health care utilization, use of medication, diagnosis, and cause of pain.[38,39] Functional limitations are measured as the effect of pain on the patient's concentration and cognitive processes, activities of daily living (ADL), emotional status, and functional abilities as perceived by the patient and physicians.[12,40,41] Employment history or vocational rehabilitation potential are assessed less frequently but are deemed important with respect to treatment outcomes.[42,43]

The wide array of areas investigated during pain assessment has necessitated the use of a variety of assessment approaches. Both the patient's perspective and the physician's perspective seem crucial in the assessment of the multiple dimensions of the patient's pain. Subjective measures such as patient self-report and physician interpretation are essential additions to the objective information obtained by the physician through a physical examination However, all instruments currently in use reflect a single approach such as the patient's subjective perspective,[44,45] the physician's subjective perspective,[15] or objective physical measurements.[39,40]

As pain treatment centers are increasing throughout the nation, a rational and consistent assessment of the areas of a person's life related to and affected by the presence of chronic pain is a growing need. The present assessment strategies, and subsequent outcomes, among the various treatment centers are not directly comparable. At present, the varied methods used at different pain treatment centers to assess the patient preclude comparison of pain treatment techniques across centers.[43,46,47] The statistical manipulations of meta-analysis procedures are being used to perform this function.[77,87] Other facilities that must evaluate factors related to chronic pain are struggling with the same concerns of noncomparability. A vital need has therefore been identified for a valid and reliable multiperspective, multidimensional pain assessment tool.[48] The use of a standardized protocol would alleviate this problem of noncomparability.

The Multiperspective Multidimensional Pain Assessment Protocol was developed to fulfill these needs. The MMPAP is a pain assessment tool that encompasses all domains previously assessed by varied means. The MMPAP was originally developed by extensive literature review and was further developed by two expert panel roundtable reviews. This process of initial development ensures that the MMPAP expands upon earlier research and addresses the shortcomings previously described. Data were collected from a variety of perspectives: The patient supplied basic demographic and vocational information on an initial referral form and completed a subjective assessment instrument containing pain information, both historical and at the time of completion. Two physicians performed a physical examination and completed a form containing both subjective and objective information plus treatment history. The comprehensive list of forced-choice items was initially pilot tested with 67 patients reporting pain for at least 6 months. Those components that could not be consistently and repeatedly assessed were dropped from the battery.

Following the initial development of the MMPAP, the protocol was validated and tested for reliability. Herein are described the research design, methodology, and results of reliability, concurrent validity, and construct validity analyses completed as components of this standardization of the MMPAP.

METHODS

Standardization of the MMPAP was a sequential process. Analyses were initially performed to ensure that the data collected were reliable across examiner and time. The internal consistency of all indices initially conceptualized was tested with Chronbach's α before using the indices in any subsequent analyses. Concurrent validity analyses were then completed to provide an assessment of the validity of the MMPAP in relation to that of previously validated assessment tools. Construct validity was then assessed as the final component in this standardization phase.

Sample
Two primary constraints were required for participation within this study: (a) the individual had to have chronic pain, strictly defined within this study to be pain of a duration of 6 months or more; and (b) the individual had to be an adult of working age and could not have taken early retirement. Working age is defined as 18 to 64 years. To perform the analyses, recruiting both employed and unemployed people on an equal basis was necessary. Every other low back pain patient randomly selected was recruited to limit the size of this large group of chronic pain patients. This selection constraint allowed us to perform the complex statistical analyses on a wide spectrum of chronic pain conditions without requiring a prohibitively large sample size.[79]

Table 7-1 Demographic Composition of the MMPAP Validity Sample (n = 651)

Demographic Description	Frequency	Percentage
Race		
Black	189	29.0
White	438	67.3
Other	24	3.7
Gender		
Male	263	40.4
Female	388	59.6
Age (y)		
Less than 40	280	43.0
40–54	303	46.5
55 and older	68	10.4

A total of 691 outpatients from various clinics at a major medical institution on the east coast initially volunteered. Thirty-six of these individuals later refused participation. Since the entire MMPAP is completed on the same day, only four patients did not complete the assessment. The entire MMPAP was therefore administered to a total of 651 outpatients, for a response rate of 94%. The length of time to complete was very patient specific, and varied from 2 to 4 hours.

All participants had chronic pain, strictly defined within this study to be pain of a duration of 6 months or more, regardless of the initial cause of the pain. All participants were adults of working age, 18 to 64 years old. To assess the related elements of those individuals who remain employed although they have pain, as well as those who are not employed, the sample was selected a priori as half employed and half unemployed. Table 7-1 summarizes key demographic information for the sample.

Development of the Protocol

A multiphase process was used to develop, standardize, and validate the pain assessment protocol. The questionnaires for this study originated with the Pain Commission suggestions for items or indicators hypothesized to be potentially helpful in pain assessment.[5] These initial items were then expanded by a team of chronic pain experts from around the country in a series of roundtable discussions to include all areas of investigation thought necessary to create a comprehensive list. The structure of the MMPAP consists of individual items combined into domains. The initial items and domains were based on expert-panel recommendations and literature review and were subsequently modified by factor analysis.

Table 7-2   Domain and Construct Descriptions

Rating of Pain Dimensions

Pain description

Psychological perception of pain

Perception of control over pain

Pain behaviors

Pain interference with sleep

Medical Information

Health care utilization

Medication/tolerance of painful medical procedures

Family history

Physical examination

Effectiveness of past treatments

Review of diagnostic evaluations and procedures

Review of medications—past and current

Mental Health

Depression

Emotional status

Contact with the mental health system

Substance abuse

Social Support Networks

Significant other support of individual with pain

Functional Limitations

Effect on concontration and cognitive processes

Effect on ADL

Effect on emotional status

Functional abilities

Employment or Rehabilitation

Rehabilitation and work potential

Motivation

Individual items were grouped into similar categories or indices, called *components.* In turn, individual components were grouped to form the major domains. Each of these domains is briefly described and is tabulated with its component constructs in Table 7-2. Because the total assessment tool is 23 pages long (see Appendices 1 through 4), sample questions that were used to assess the domains are provided in an effort to illustrate the actual assessment instrument.

The rating of pain dimensions domain includes pain description items such as frequency, duration, intensity and unpleasantness, psychological perception of pain, pain behaviors, perception of control over pain, and pain interference with sleep. This information is collected through patient reports (Table 7-3) and physician ratings (Table 7-4).

The mental health status domain includes the patient's self-report of depressive symptoms, contact with the mental health system, substance abuse, and sociopathy (Table 7-5). This domain also includes the physician's perception of patient depression, substance abuse, and other mental health indicators.

The social support network domain includes the patient's perception of support provided by his or her significant other, the patient's perception of the significant other's reaction to the patient, and each physician's perception of the patient's social support network.

The medical information domain is primarily a series of questions related to the two independent physical examinations. It also includes health care utilization, use of medication, and willingness to tolerate painful medical procedures, as collected through patient reports and physician ratings, diagnostic testing, diagnosis, and cause of pain.

The functional limitations domain includes an assessment of the effect of pain on the patient's concentration and cognitive processes, ADL, emotional status, and functional abilities as perceived by the patient and physicians. The employment or rehabilitation potential domain contains the perceptions of the physicians regarding the patient's employment potential and motivation to work (Table 7-6).

Data Collection

Data were collected from a variety of perspectives. The patients supplied basic demographic and vocational information on a referral form and completed an additional patient self-reporting instrument that contained pain information, both historical and at the time of assessment. The patient provided an assessment of history, location, frequency, duration, severity, and intensity of pain with exacerbating factors; history of health care use for diagnosis and treatment of pain (i.e., surgical, pharmaceutical, physician visits, hospitalizations); current usage and future need for health care; pain behaviors prior to and since the onset of pain; cognitive status and ability for task completion; emotional disturbance prior to and since the onset of pain; history of mental health intervention; ADL and social functioning prior to and since the onset of pain; and functional ability and limitations. All items were forced choice with a continuous 5- or 6-point scale whenever possible. Table 7-7 identifies the perspectives with respect to each domain on the MMPAP.

Two physicians completed a full physical examination using a standard protocol in which similar specified detailed examination

Table 7-3 Sample of Claimant Rating of Pain Dimensions

Question	Rating
In the past 6 months, how often have you had pain?	1 = Less than once a month 2 = At least once a month 3 = At least once a week 4 = At least once a day 5 = Several times per day to continuously
If you have had pain-free periods in the past 6 months, how long do they usually last?	0 = No pain-free periods 1 = Minutes 2 = Hours 3 = Days 4 = Weeks 5 = Months
In the past 6 months, when have you had pain? How long has the pain usually lasted?	1 = 5 min or less 2 = Over 5 min to 1 h 3 = Over 1 h to 1 day 4 = Over 1 day to 1 week 5 = Over 1 week to continuously
In the past 6 months, at what time of day has your pain been the worst?	1 = Always the same level of severity 2 = When you first get up 3 = Morning 4 = Afternoon 5 = Evening 6 = Right before bedtime 7 = At night, when you are trying to sleep 8 = Gets worse and better, but no specific pattern 9 = Both morning and evening
In the past 6 months, how often has the pain made it hard to get to sleep?	1 = Not at all 2 = Some nights 3 = Most nights 4 = Almost every night 5 = Every night
In the past 6 months, how often has the pain awakened you from sleep?	1 = Not at all 2 = Some nights 3 = Most nights 4 = Almost every night 5 = Every night
How difficult is it to put up with or cope with your pain?	1 = Easy 2 = Inconvenient 3 = Troublesome 4 = Very difficult 5 = Almost impossible
How much does the pain interfere with what you want to do?	1 = No restrictions 2 = Minor interference 3 = Moderate obstacle 4 = A great barrier 5 = Hinders all activities

Table 7-4   Sample of Physician Rating of Pain Dimensions

Question	Rating	
To what degree has the patient		
displayed pain behavior signs (e.g., grimacing, shifting, audible indications)?	1 = None 2 = Slight 3 = Moderate	4 = Marked 5 = Extreme 6 = IE
talked about pain?	1 = None 2 = Slight 3 = Moderate	4 = Marked 5 = Extreme 6 = IE
displayed abnormal posturing or abnormal movement due to pain?	1 = None 2 = Slight 3 = Moderate	4 = Marked 5 = Extreme 6 = IE
experienced sleep disturbances due to pain?	1 = None 2 = Slight 3 = Moderate	4 = Marked 5 = Extreme 6 = IE
exhibited more mood alterations than other patients with similar problems?	1 = None 2 = Slight 3 = Moderate	4 = Marked 5 = Extreme 6 = IE
utilized health care services compared with patients with similar problems?	1 = None 2 = Slight 3 = Moderate	4 = Marked 5 = Extreme 6 = IE
been compliant with prescribed care?	1 = None 2 = Slight 3 = Moderate	4 = Marked 5 = Extreme 6 = IE
expressed willingness to undergo repeated painful diagnostic procedures or surgery?	1 = None 2 = Slight 3 = Moderate	4 = Marked 5 = Extreme 6 = IE

IE, insufficient evidence.

techniques and parameters were used for all assessments. The protocol precluded the physician from asking the patient to repeat a personal answer to the questions that were on the patient questionnaire but instead required the physician to give an independent assessment of the items. During the examination the physician was permitted to ask a variety of open-ended questions to assist in this endeavor. The protocol included the physician's evaluation of the following patient characteristics: pain complaint, including sensory and affective intensity; frequency and duration of pain; utilization of health care systems; exhibitions of pain behaviors; emotional status; cognitive and functional status; ability to complete a task; physical examination including range of motion, neurological examination, vascular examination, assessment of trigger points and tender points, assessment of magnification or exaggeration of symptoms, and specific evidence of physical impairment; laboratory and imaging data supporting the patient's pain complaint: and functional ability and rehabilitation potential. All items were forced choice with a continuous 5- and

Table 7-5   Sample of Claimant Rating of Mental Health Status

Question	Rating	
In the *past week*, how often have you felt that		
you will always have health problems?	1 = Always 2 = Most times 3 = Often	4 = Sometimes 5 = Never
your situation is hopeless?	1 = Always 2 = Most times 3 = Often	4 = Sometimes 5 = Never
you will never be able to work again?	1 = Always 2 = Most times 3 = Often	4 = Sometimes 5 = Never
you will never be able to do things you used to enjoy?	1 = Always 2 = Most times 3 = Often	4 = Sometimes 5 = Never
you have no motivation to get better?	1 = Always 2 = Most times 3 = Often	4 = Sometimes 5 = Never

Question	Frequency	Severity
In the past 6 months, how frequently and severely did you feel		
depressed?	0 = Never 1 = Sometimes 2 = Often	1 = Mildly 2 = Moderately 3 = Severely
frustrated?	0 = Never 1 = Sometimes 2 = Often	1 = Mildly 2 = Moderately 3 = Severely
anxious?	0 = Never 1 = Sometimes 2 = Often	1 = Mildly 2 = Moderately 3 = Severely
angry?	0 = Never 1 = Sometimes 2 = Often	1 = Mildly 2 = Moderately 3 = Severely
guilty?	0 = Never 1 = Sometimes 2 = Often	1 = Mildly 2 = Moderately 3 = Severely

6-point scale whenever possible. The treating physician also completed a historical section outlining previous services, treatments, and medications.

Rater Reliability

Rater reliability, both test-retest and interrater, was assessed to ensure that the MMPAP provided consistent information. Twenty percent of the participating patients were randomly selected for a second recruitment to again undergo the battery of assessments for reliability analyses.

Table 7-6 Sample of Physicians' Rating of Employment or Rehabilitation Potential

Question	Rating
Which of the following definitions best describe the patient's pain situation?	1 = Patient does not have chronic pain 2 = Chronic pain, inability to cope; insufficient documented impairment 3 = Chronic pain, competent coping; insufficient documented impairment 4 = Chronic pain, inability to cope; documented impairment sufficient 5 = Chronic pain, competent coping; documented impairment sufficient
Did the patient react appropriately to the exam, or did the pain behaviors appear exaggerated?	1 = Appropriate response 2 = Exaggerated response
In your estimation, how supportive is the patient's social support network in terms of providing emotional support and practical assistance that will enable the patient to effectively cope with the pain (e.g., significant other, family, friends)?	1 = Very supportive 2 = Somewhat supportive 3 = Ambivalent 4 = Somewhat critical or unsympathetic 5 = Intolerant
If this patient had a sufficient support system (e.g., a very supportive family or significant other), how good a candidate do you believe he/she would be for participation in a rehabilitation program?	1 = Excellent 2 = Good 3 = Average 4 = Poor 5 = Definitely not a candidate 6 = Does not need
How motivated do you believe this patient has been or would be in terms of changing his/her lifestyle (e.g., lower pay, move, take a less desirable job) in order to be rehabilitated?	1 = Extremely motivated 2 = Moderately motivated 3 = Somewhat motivated 4 = Slightly motivated 5 = Not motivated
To what extent are the pain complaints greater than would be expected from objective clinical findings?	1 = No greater 2 = Slight 3 = Moderate 4 = Marked 5 = Extreme 6 = IE
In your opinion, will the patient require more, less, or the same level of treatment in the next year?	1 = Less 2 = Same 3 = More

IE, insufficient evidence.

Rater reliability refers to the extent to which measurement error is created either by implementation of a questionnaire from one time to another or by implementation of the same instrument by a different administrator. In the second assessment visit, care was taken either to match patients with physicians and nurses who had assessed them previously (test-retest reliability) or to mix patients with different sets of clinical researchers (interrater reliability).

Table 7-7   Domain Assessment Perspectives

Domain	Perspective
Rating of pain dimensions	Patient self-report Physician assessment
Medical information	Patient self-report Physical examination Physician assessment
Mental health	Patient self-report Physician assessment
Social support networks	Patient self-report Physician assessment
Functional limitations	Patient self-report Physical examination Physician assessment
Employment or rehabilitation	Physician assessment

A total of 99 patients were examined twice and completed two sets of instruments. They were chosen randomly and were demographically similar to the entire sample. The second assessment was completed an average of 31 days after the first. Cohen's κ rater reliability was used.[83] For variables with continuous or scaled (Likert) response options, a weighted Cohen's κ was used to accommodate possible scaled chance agreement. Cohen's κ is a highly conservative reliability statistic that takes into account chance agreement, making a κ score of 0.60 roughly functionally equivalent to a Pearson's score of 0.90.[83]

Index Reliability

Index reliability refers to the extent to which each domain within each instrument, as well as the constructs within the domains, have internal consistency. The index reliability was performed using all 651 patients. Components of the indices include the continuously scaled (Likert response) and appropriate yes/no response questions. For each domain and its specific constructs, an index is created within a specific instrument only if two or more scaled items represent the domain or construct within the instrument. A high index reliability ensures the use of such indices with confidence that the questions within the index are sufficiently related to each other, allowing analyses to be performed on the index rather than individual variables. Therefore, a high index reliability shows good internal consistency for the index in question.

The Chronbach's α item analysis is the universally accepted statistic for index reliability and was performed upon each related group of questions, or index, within each instrument (e.g., all the mental health questions on the form). The target rate for index reliability, called the α score, was an internal consistency of 0.70. Domains and constructs with a lower index reliability were examined, and questions that seemed inconsistent with the others in the domain category were removed or placed into more appropriate domains.

Concurrent Validity

Concurrent validity analyses were completed to provide an assessment of the validity of the MMPAP in relation to previously validated assessment tools. Although it is generally acknowledged that pain is a multidimensional experience, currently no single comprehensive pain assessment instrument is available. No instruments presently in use for the assessment of chronic pain patients span the breadth of the MMPAP. Several standardized instruments that focus on specific aspects of the pain experience were used to assess the concurrent validity of corresponding indices of the MMPAP:

> Center for Epidemiological Studies Depression Scale (CES-D)
> Family Adaptability & Cohesion Evaluation Score: Couple Version (FACES III)
> Multidimensional Pain Instrument (MPI)
> McGill Pain Questionnaire (MPQ)
> Oswestry, Shropshire Low Back Pain Assessment (Oswestry)
> Summary of Nonorganic Physical Signs in Low Back Pain (Waddell)

Pearson correlation analyses were performed between appropriate indices on the MMPAP and related indices on each of these forms. Significant correlations show that the forms measure related constructs. Each of the concurrent validity forms used is described briefly.

CES-D

The CES-D scale is designed to provide an index of the number and frequency of depressive symptoms a person may experience in a given week.[34] It contains 20 items that are statements of how the individual felt or behaved. A person is then asked to rate the frequency of occurrence of each feeling or behavior from 1 to 7 days. The CES-D possesses internal consistency across diverse population subgroups and has a relatively good short-term test-retest reliability.[71–73] The CES-D has been used concurrently in many studies and has been shown to have a high factorial validity.[71]

FACES III

The FACES III: Couple Version consists of 10 questions that ask the person to describe his or her family at the present time, using a 5-point continuous scale. This scale contains 10 items that identify cohesion and 10 items that identify adaptability. Two items compose each of the following five concepts related to the cohesion dimension: emotional bonding, supportiveness, family boundaries, time and friendship, and interest in recreation. There are also two items for each concept related to the adaptability dimension: leadership, control, and discipline. Four items are included that combine the concepts of roles and rules.[70]

MPI

The MPI is an assessment divided into three parts with 13 empirically derived scales. Part I contains five scales designed to assess chronic pain patients: reports of pain severity, perceptions of how pain interferes with their lives, appraisals of how much support is received from significant others, perceived life control, and affective distress. Part II contains the frequency of a range of behavioral responses by significant others to their display of pain. This 14-question section can be broken into three smaller scales: punishing responses, solicitous responses, and distracting responses. Part III is an activity checklist that contains 19 common activities used to form a general activity scale, which is also divided into five smaller scales: household chores, outdoor work, activities away from home, social activities, and general activity level. The pain classification system employed in the MPI has been shown by Turk and colleagues[29] and by subsequent researchers[67] to have a good reliability and external validity.

MPQ

The MPQ is a tool that elicits three types of measures of pain, including (a) the pain rating index based on the rank values of the words that add up to a score for each category, (b) the number of words chosen by the patient, and (c) the word combination chosen as the indicator of overall pain intensity at the time the questionnaire is administered.[28] Variable reliability has been reported for the MPQ and its subscales.[28,60,61]

Oswestry

The Oswestry is a questionnaire designed to assess the effects of low back and leg pain on daily living.[15] The questionnaire is divided into 10 questions outlining different dimensions of living daily with pain: pain intensity, personal care, lifting, walking, sitting, standing, sleeping, sex life, social life, and traveling. The utility of the Oswestry has been documented by its widespread clinical use.[15,68,69]

Waddell

The Waddell Summary of Nonorganic Physical Signs in Low Back Pain is a standardized group of five types of physical signs that patients with low back pain may display. These signs are tenderness (superficial or nonanatomic), simulation (axial loading or rotation), distraction (straight leg raising), regional (weakness or sensory), and overreaction. The form is completed by the examining physician. A finding of three or more of the five types of signs is considered clinically significant. Waddell initially validated this instrument through four studies conducted in Canada, Scotland, and Great Britain.[39]

The concurrent validity phase of the study ensured two critical conditions. First, it assured that the concurrent validity of the MMPAP was tested with statistically appropriate groups. Second, it ensured that the pain assessment protocol had been shown to have high correlations with reliable, valid, and currently used instruments in the field. These and subsequent analyses were conducted to increase the efficiency and economy of instrument clinical use.

Construct Validity

To assess the construct validity of the MMPAP, principal factor analysis with varimax rotation of factors was performed on the protocol responses. The basic notion behind the application of factor analysis is that a higher-order (i.e., not directly measurable) factor is composed, in some part, of measurable outwardly manifested behaviors or actions. Construct validity is an indication of the degree to which a set of measurements of related variables actually approaches the measurement of the hypothesized construct.[84] The factor analysis generates *loadings* or weights for all components of each extracted factor. Items with high loadings for a factor explain some component of variation for that factor.

Principal-factor analysis is the most commonly used statistic in construct validity analysis.[88] With this approach, selected indices consist of related questions within a group and are parts of components or domains. Items with high loadings for a factor explain some component of variation for that factor. Prior to analysis, all scaled items were ordered from positive to negative (i.e., all items that began with negative options were reversed). Questions relating to the patient's experiences before the onset of pain were inappropriate for factor analysis because of the time frame and therefore were excluded from analysis. Although all generated factors were reviewed, only factors with eigen values approaching 1.0 or greater were retained in the final analysis. To confirm the adequacy of the sample size for this factor analysis, Kaiser's measure of sampling adequacy[85] was performed on all factor samples.

Since it was anticipated that the patient's responses would be correlated with the physicians' responses, two independent analyses were performed. The resulting factors within an analysis were uncorrelated. Although individual perspective analyses create distinct models, the same domains are assessed within each perspective. Therefore, although combining the instruments for analyses is appropriate on the domain level or at least on the construct level, it is not appropriate on the item level.

RESULTS

Rater Reliability

The overall rater reliability of the patient perspective scored above the target level of 0.60 with an interrater reliability of 0.61 (n = 35) and a

Table 7-8   Rater Reliability Scores

Domain	Test-Retest (same test administrator)	Interrater (different test administrator)
Patient perspective (total)	0.63	0.61
Rating of pain dimensions	0.62	0.58
Medical information	0.69	0.71
Mental health	0.71	0.62
Social support networks	0.51	0.48
Functional limitations	0.56	0.54
Physician perspective (total)	0.70	0.61
Rating of pain dimensions	0.83	0.75
Medical information	0.67	0.62
Mental health	0.79	0.52
Social support networks	0.74	0.50
Functional limitations	0.75	0.68

Cohen's κ and weighted Cohen's κ were used for all tests.

test-retest reliability of 0.63 (n = 64) (Table 7-8). Although most of the domains scored consistently well, several questions exploring the patient's emotions (i.e., calm, frustrated, anxious, angry) had relatively low rater reliability scores, reducing the entire reliability. The final reliability scores from the physicians' perspective after deletion or modification of low rater reliability variables are 0.70 for test-retest and 0.61 for interrater (see Table 7-8). A number of individual items, most unrelated to patient medical history, were noted to have low rater reliability scores. The social support domain was removed from the later construct validity analysis because all three questions on the physician instruments that related to social support had a low rater reliability.

Index Reliability
The index reliability of each domain of the patient perspective was high; there were satisfactory index reliability scores for the component constructs. Although the contact with the mental health system construct under the mental health domain was quite low with an index reliability of 0.54, the domain had a reliability of 0.82. The health care utilization construct reliability (0.69) and the medication and willingness to tolerate painful medical procedures construct reliability (0.66) were also less than 0.70. However, the encompassing domain, medical information, had the sizable index reliability of 0.81, allowing analyses to be performed using this domain (Table 7-9).

The domain reliability scores and most construct reliability scores were quite high for the physician's perspective. Several isolated

Table 7-9 Patient Perspective Domain and Item Analyses

Domain	α Score
Rating of pain dimensions	0.94
Pain description	0.92
Psychological perception of pain	0.90
Perception of control over pain	0.71
Pain interference with sleep	0.82
Medical information	0.81
Health care utilization	0.69
Medication/tolerance of painful medical procedures	0.66
Family history	0.81
Mental health	0.82
Depression	0.85
Contact with the mental health system	0.54
Substance abuse	0.89
Social support networks	0.79
Significant other support of individual with pain	0.79
Functional limitations	0.93
Effect on concentration and cognitive processes	0.74
Effect on ADL	0.83
Effect on emotional status	0.88
Functional abilities	0.85

constructs had considerably lower α reliability scores. The index components are consequently designed for use in analyses as individual variables or as components of indices that span perspectives. Because all domain reliability scores were well above 0.70, no additional items were deleted on the basis of this analysis (Table 7-10).

Concurrent Validity

As noted previously, no single currently available comprehensive pain assessment tool spans the breadth and depth of the MMPAP. The MPQ and the MPI are currently the most widely used multidimensional assessment instruments. These instruments, along with several standardized instruments widely used in the study of pain, were used to assess concurrent validity of the MMPAP. The additional instruments used were the CES-D, the FACES III, the Oswestry, and the Waddell.

Each concurrent validity instrument was administered with the main protocol to a random sample of patients; sample sizes ranged from 55 to 199, depending on the size of the instrument. Larger instruments required larger sample sizes for analysis. The sample size varied slightly between indices on an instrument, mainly because some questions, notably the sex or spousal/social interactions questions on the MPI and the Oswestry, were not applicable to all respondents. The demographic compositions of these subsamples were comparable with the composition of the entire sample. Results of these analyses are enumerated in Table 7-11.

Table 7-10   Physician Perspective Domain and Item Analyses

Domain	α Score
Rating of pain dimensions	0.83
Pain description	0.68
Rating of pain behaviors	0.81
Rating of pain interference with sleep	0.88
Medical information	0.80
Perception of patient's willingness to tolerate painful medical procedures and overuse of health care systems	0.63
Physical examination	0.82
Effectiveness of past treatments	0.83
Review of all diagnostic evaluations and procedures	0.72
Review of all medications—past and current	0.62
Mental health	0.88
Perceptions of patient's emotional status	0.88
Perception of patient's mental health	0.82
Perception of patient's substance abuse	0.52
Social support networks	0.90
Perception of patient's social support network	0.90
Functional limitations	0.97
Perception of effect on concentration and cognition	0.82
Perception of effect on ADL and personal interactions	0.92
Perception of patient's functional abilities	0.97
Employment	0.81
Perception of patient's rehabilitation and work potential	0.78
Perception of patient's motivation	0.82

CES-D

The CES-D was administered to a random sample of 199 patients with the MMPAP. Concurrent validity was assessed between the CES-D and an index on the MMPAP that consisted of affective and depression questions throughout the patient's component of the MMPAP. This index, which had an internal consistency of 0.93, had a highly significant correlation with the CES-D (see Table 7-11).

FACES III

The FACES III: Couples Version was administered to a random sample of 56 married patients with the MMPAP. Each spouse also completed a FACES III. Concurrent validity was assessed between the FACES III and two indices on the MMPAP. The first index was a group of spouse interaction items that the patient completed. This index, which had an internal consistency of 0.73, had a statistically significant moderate correlation with the patient FACES III (see Table 7-11). The second index was a group of spouse interaction questions that the patient's significant other completed. This index, which had an internal consistency of 0.63, had a highly significant correlation with the significant other FACES III (see Table 7-11).

Table 7-11 Concurrent Validity Analyses between Previously Validated Instruments and Related Indices of the MMPAP

Instrument	Index	n	Correlation Coefficient	Significance Level
CES-D	—	199	0.80	.0001
FACES III	Patient	56	0.31	.0204
	Significant other	51	0.60	.0001
MPI	Pain	129	0.73	.0001
	Interference	104	0.55	.0001
	Life control	133	0.41	.0001
	Affective distress	129	0.21	.0149
	Support	129	0.33	.0001
	Punishing responses	110	0.34	.0003
	Solicitous responses	129	0.51	.0001
	Distracting responses	129	0.42	.0001
	Household chores	108	0.62	.0001
	Outdoor work	109	0.23	.0158
	Activities from home	109	0.24	.0131
	Social activities	110	0.21	.0282
	General activity	133	0.34	.0001
MPQ	—	97	0.43	.0001
Oswestry	Functional limitations	117	0.71	.0001
	Sex	67	0.52	.0001
	Sleep	106	0.58	.0001
	Pain	104	0.42	.0001
	ADL	67	0.50	.0001
Waddell	—	55	0.67	.0001

MPI

The MPI was administered to a random sample of 133 patients with the MMPAP. Concurrent validity was assessed between the 13 scales on the MPI and 13 corresponding indices on the MMPAP. All correlations were significant, ranging from a low of 0.21 for the social activities subscale to 0.73 for the pain-related questions index (see Table 7-11).

MPQ

The MPQ was administered to a random sample of 97 patients with the MMPAP. Concurrent validity was assessed between the MPQ Pain Rating Index (PRI) and one index on the MMPAP. The index consisted of pain-related questions throughout the MMPAP. Results showed that this index had a statistically significant moderate correlation with the MPQ (see Table 7-11).

Oswestry

The Oswestry was administered to a random sample of 117 patients with a primary complaint of back or leg pain with the MMPAP. Concurrent validity was assessed between different sections of the

Oswestry and five indices on the MMPAP. The functional limitations index had a highly significant correlation with Oswestry questions 3 through 6 (see Table 7-11). The sex-related questions index, which had an internal consistency of 0.72, had a highly significant correlation with Oswestry question 8. The sleep-related questions index, which had an internal consistency of 0.87, had a highly significant correlation with Oswestry question 7. The pain-related questions index, which had an internal consistency of 0.97, had a significant correlation with Oswestry question 1. The ADL questions, which had an internal consistency of 0.90, had a highly significant correlation with Oswestry questions 2, 9, and 10 (see Table 7-11).

Waddell
The Waddell was completed by those physicians who examined a random sample of 55 patients with a primary complaint of low back pain. Concurrent validity was assessed between the Waddell and the MMPAP items addressing functional capacity evaluation (FCE) level of effort and symptom exaggeration questions from the physicians' perspective. This index, which had an internal consistency of 0.77, had a highly significant correlation with the Waddell (see Table 7-11).

Construct Validity
Although 651 patients completed the reliability and validity phase of the pain assessment study, missing information reduced the effective sample size of these analyses to 637 without demographic deviations from the larger sample. A principal factor analysis was performed on the domains listed earlier with varimax rotation of factors. Although additional factors were reviewed, only those factors with eigen values near 1.0 or greater were retained in the final analysis. Kaiser's measure of sampling adequacy was sufficient for all analyses with a value of 0.93 for the patient's perspective and a value of 0.89 for the physicians' perspective.

Patient
Twelve factors were retained by the factor analysis of the patient's perspective (Table 7-12). The first factor contained pain descriptors about intensity and unpleasantness and an item concerning coping skills. The second factor highlighted functional abilities, such as lifting items from floor to counter. The third factor contained ADL items.

The fourth factor included additional ADL but also contained questions related to ADL, such as items related to activity environment (e.g., temperature) or physical activity (e.g., walking). The fifth factor consisted of items reflecting mood alteration. The sixth factor contained items that described the patient's emotional outlook. Family history would describe the items included in the seventh factor. Factor 8 pertained to the actions of the significant other, such as offering assistance. The ninth factor consisted of items that describe the effect of pain on the patient's cognitive ability, including memory.

Table 7-12   Patient Perspective: Variance Explained by Each Factor

Factor Number and Description	Eigen Value
1. Pain descriptions	5.81
2. Functional abilities	5.10
3. Effects on ADL	4.66
4. Environmental components	4.45
5. Mood alteration	4.27
6. Emotional descriptors	3.35
7. Family history	2.76
8. Significant other actions	2.76
9. Effect on cognitive processes	2.43
10. Functional repetitions	2.19
11. Significant other reactions	1.84
12. Pain interference with sleep	1.17

Factor 10 dealt with strenuous repeated activity (such as reaching and squatting). Factor 11 suggested the significant other's emotional reaction to the patient, and factor 12 encompassed sleep disturbance issues.

Some domains clustered appropriately, but the factors they comprised did not contribute significantly to the overall variance. The entirety of the mental health status domain had low loadings. Pain behavior and a motivation question also loaded low, as did job completion, sexual difficulties, and eating disorders. Although these items remain in the protocol, they are not recognized as independent factors.

Physician

A total of eight factors was retained by the physicians' perspective factor analysis (Table 7-13). The first factor was primarily a functional activities factor with conditional restrictions such as heat and cold. This factor also contained an indicator of whether the patient can work full-time and an indicator of the frequency of pain. The second factor was related to motivation for employment, including items from both the employment domain and the social support domain. The third factor was a combination of subjective items from several domains. All items in this factor related to the physicians' perception of the patient's emotions, relationships, and ADL.

The fourth factor contained the medical procedure construct of the medical information domain. The fifth factor consisted of the musculoskeletal construct of the medical information domain, while the sixth factor contained the autonomic and vascular information from the medical information domain. The seventh factor consisted of descriptors related to the intensity and unpleasantness of pain. The

Table 7-13 Physician Perspective: Variance Explained by Each Factor

Factor Number and Description	Eigen Value
1. Perception of functional abilities/restrictions	4.68
2. Motivation, causes, and effects	3.03
3. Effects on emotional status/cognitive processes	2.96
4. Treatment modalities	1.51
5. Musculoskeletal indicators	1.51
6. Autonomic and vascular indicators	1.41
7. Pain descriptors	1.31
8. Tenderness and spasms	1.17

eighth factor focused on the tenderness to palpation and muscle spasm information. Medications and questions concerning compliance with prescribed care and medicinal effectiveness as well as the two questions concerning future rehabilitation predictions did not load appreciably on the eight main factors.

DISCUSSION

The MMPAP is a lengthy instrument that may require 2 hours or more to complete. It compels the administrator to obtain information from a variety of sources, including the subjective perceptions of the patient, medical record review, direct physical examination, and physician appraisal of patient behavior. Although validation analyses indicate that the instrument is effective in predicting the likelihood that an individual will return to work, the instrument is not appropriate in situations in which a quick screening tool is required.

The very factors that make the MMPAP inappropriate for use in some situations also are its major strengths. The instrument attempts to measure reliably all the major constructs viewed as important in the diagnosis or treatment of chronic pain. As a result, it necessarily focuses on information that can be obtained only through multiple perspectives—patients' and physicians'—and examines that information in sufficient detail to ensure statistical validity.

Despite its length and complexity, the MMPAP may have substantial clinical utility for a variety of purposes. First, the MMPAP was designed to assist in the disability determination process and the prediction of return to work.[89] The factors that affect the likelihood that an individual with chronic pain will enter or return to the workforce are varied and multifarious. The ability of the MMPAP to measure reliably the complex physical, psychological, and social factors that contribute to employment may make the instrument clinically appropriate in situations in which other instruments fail to measure all relevant constructs.

Second, in many situations, clinicians may already be using a variety of shorter instruments that taken as a whole may compose an informal battery that is larger and takes longer to administer than the MMPAP. For example, in some situations, clinicians may administer an instrument that examines multiple pain dimensions, another that addresses mental health factors, and a third that examines social support factors. These instruments may then be supplemented by record reviews and physical examinations. In these instances, the combined length of time involved in administering these various instruments and examinations may be equal to or greater than that for the MMPAP. The MMPAP has the advantage of standardizing and validating this process and eliminating some of the shortcomings resulting from a haphazard or informal approach.

Chronic pain has always presented a challenge to physicians in definition, classification, diagnosis, and treatment. The responsibility of physicians to detect permanent impairment and to provide recommendations regarding likelihood of returning to work is made more difficult by the complexities presented by the chronic pain patient. For physicians to address the needs of the patient with respect to treatment strategies, information must be obtained from a variety of areas. These areas include mental health status, coping mechanisms, social supports network, functional limitations and performance, rehabilitation potential, and other factors. The variety of previously described methods used at different pain treatment centers to assess the patients precludes comparison of pain treatment techniques across centers. The utilization of a standardized protocol would alleviate this problem and allow comparison of the various techniques among as well as within centers.

The assessment protocol described in this study was developed and validated under contract from the Social Security Administration. The MMPAP addresses the concerns raised in the reports by the Commission on Evaluation of Pain and the Institute of Medicine Committee Report on Pain and Disability. The MMPAP was first developed by a comprehensive literature review combined with the participation of an expert panel. The protocol was pilot tested on an independent sample of individuals with chronic pain before the present reliability and validation phase. A total of 651 patients with chronic pain completed the reliability and validity phase of the pain assessment study.

Although the sample was randomly selected from individuals presenting at a major medical institution with pain, the demographic distribution was very inclusive. Approximately two thirds of the sample was white, a little less than one third African-American, and approximately 4% consisted of individuals from other ethnic backgrounds. A significant χ^2 analysis between gender and diagnosis, with diagnosis being either low back pain or other diagnoses, supported the hypothesis that the slightly higher representation of females, at 60%, was partially caused by the deliberate suppression of the percentage of low back pain patients in the sample. Every other low back pain patient had been screened out of recruitment to limit randomly the size of this large group of chronic pain patients, allowing the representation of a wide spectrum of chronic pain conditions without requiring a prohibitively large sample size. Missing information reduced the effective sample size of some of the more comprehensive analyses to 637, but no demographic deviations from the larger sample were detected, making this a very robust sample for the rigorous validation analyses.

The overall rater reliability of the instruments was satisfactory, from both the patient's perspective and the physicians' perspective. Several questions inquiring about the patient's emotions (i.e., calm, frustrated, anxious, angry) had relatively low rater reliability scores, especially concerning pre-pain status. As these are quite often transient emotions, it is expected that these individual items would have a lower stability across a 3-week period. Also, a number of individual items, most unrelated to patient medical history, were noted to have low rater reliability scores. These reduced reliability scores were dealt with on an item-by-item basis, some related variables being combined, to allow one of the similar variables to remain in the analyses, and others being eliminated. These modifications improved the utility of the protocol as the type of data collected increased in reliability.

The index reliability of each domain of the patient perspective is high, with satisfactory index reliability scores for the component constructs. The domain reliability scores and most construct reliability scores are also quite high for the physicians' perspective. The high degree of index reliability provides additional assurance that all items within an index, which are conceptualized as related, truly do have a significant positive correlation or relationship with other items within the index.

Significant correlations were obtained between the MMPAP and all components of the currently used assessment tools, showing that the MMPAP covers the critical components addressed by each of the related instruments. This result was anticipated, since previous research on the MPI and MPQ and other instruments was heavily relied upon to develop domains contained within the MMPAP. This is also true for the mental health and social support indicators, for which a high concurrent validity was obtained between relevant indices of the MMPAP and both the CES-D and the FACES III.

The high concurrent validity between the physical examination component of the MMPAP and the two physician instruments, the Oswestry and the Waddell, was less expected. Physicians within private practice routinely order functional performance evaluations of their new chronic pain patients. However, when a standard protocol is followed for the physical examination, the physician is apparently able to estimate accurately the patient's functional abilities and limitations and anticipate standard responses to the nonorganic physical signs tests.

The 12 factors retained by the principal-factor analysis of the patient perspective and also the eight factors retained by the physician factor analysis lent credence to the originally conceptualized domains. It was anticipated that there would be one general pain description factor for each perspective, with several smaller factors that would correspond to the domains. The first factor of the patient's perspective was indeed pain descriptors, specifically related to intensity, unpleasantness, and coping. However, there was a fairly even distribution of factors rather than one large overriding factor. The evenly distributed eigen values across factors that quite accurately delineate the originally conceptualized domains lend credence to the assertion that distinct domains are being accurately measured.

Functional ability was prominent in both analyses as the second factor from the patient's perspective and the first factor of the physicians' perspective. ADL dominated the subsequent two factors of the patient's perspective and the third factor of the physicians' perspective. The second factor of the physicians' perspective appeared to be related to motivation, and it contained items from two domains— employment and social support. The physical examination portion of the protocol grouped by related items to form the fourth, fifth, sixth, and eighth factors of the physicians' perspective. Questions from the medical information domain concerning medical testing, medical visits, medications, and family history had low loadings for the patients' perspective, which emphasizes the necessity of both perspectives in a comprehensive protocol.

Implications of the Study
Taken in concert, the reliability and validation analyses show that the MMPAP is a concise, repeatable, and valid assessment of the major domains related to chronic pain. Utilization of a standardized assessment will aid in consistent diagnosis and treatment both within and across pain treatment centers. The results of the validation analysis indicated that the MMPAP is a valid clinical tool when administered by physicians trained in the use of the protocol. The reliability analyses confirmed that stable constructs are measured, showing that individual responses do not fluctuate significantly within a 3-week period, with the same or different administrators. Clinical utility is enhanced by the fact that the MMPAP does not require expensive or specialized equipment but is simply a structured multidimensional examination and self-report questionnaire.

Using a comprehensive standardized assessment protocol can aid in early identification of problems in the psychological, vocational, functional, or behavioral areas that might not be apparent until later in traditional assessment and treatment processes. Identification of problems with a valid and reliable standardized assessment protocol would also be helpful for the patient and physician when dealing with insurance companies and workers compensation claims.

The significant correlations obtained between the MMPAP and all components of the currently used assessment tools indicated that the MMPAP covers the critical components addressed by each of the related instruments. Of course, the primary advantage of the MMPAP over these other instruments that assess the same domains is that with the MMPAP, they are all assessed within the same protocol. The adoption of this protocol as the standard would allow direct comparison of pain treatment efficacy across pain treatment centers.

The protocol could also be used in studies investigating the relative efficacy of various rehabilitation interventions. As with the development of any comprehensive assessment tool, some information was retained on the protocol because it was deemed helpful by the physicians to maintain a thorough assessment. Utilization of this protocol with chronic pain patients should give the clinician the ability to assess chronic pain accurately and consistently early in the medical evaluation and treatment plan, which could influence the choices of a treatment plan. For example, patients could receive psychological, vocational, comprehensive rehabilitation or behavioral interventions earlier. The use of appropriate clinical interventions earlier in the process would undoubtedly improve clinical outcomes. Identification of patients with chronic pain with a valid and reliable instrument could help in finding interventions that lessen or alleviate the pain or change other pain-related outcomes.

SUMMARY

A major need identified by the Commission on Evaluation of Pain, the Institute of Medicine, and the SSA has been for a valid, reliable multi-dimensional assessment tool for the patient with chronic pain. The great need for a rational and consistent decision-making process concerning chronic pain and disability is apparent. Inconsistencies exist in physical examinations, history-taking techniques, and interpretation of examination and history findings for chronic pain. In this time of limited resources and of increasing expectations, decisions regarding resources for chronic pain patients (disability benefits; access to pain treatment centers, rehabilitation, etc.) must be made and are being made on a daily basis. Physicians are being asked by workers compensation carriers, federal agencies, and the judiciary system to provide information and recommendations. These groups have varying levels of training, knowledge, and experience about pain and disability. In the past there has not been a consistent or rational data collection process to support or guide the decisions. These decisions ultimately affect psychosocial, physical, and economic aspects of patients' lives, as well as the economics of business, industry, and government.

The implications of the development of this standardized protocol are far ranging. The MMPAP has potential as a diagnostic tool as well as a measure of treatment effectiveness. Utilization of the MMPAP will allow the comparison of various pain treatment center outcomes. The MMPAP has been proved to be a valid and reliable pain assessment protocol that encompasses all domains related to chronic pain assessment within one multiperspective tool. Additional research is needed to confirm and extend the results of the present investigation. Research possibilities are to demonstrate the therapeutic and diagnostic utility of the protocol in a way that could perhaps improve the various agencies' and organizations' responsiveness and decisions affecting individuals with chronic pain.

References

1. Bostrom M. Summary of the Mayday Fund Survey: public attitudes about pain and analgesics. *J Pain Symptom Manage.* 1997; 13:166–168.
2. Osterweis M, Kleinman A, Mechanic D, eds. *Pain and Disability: Clinical, Behavioral, and Public Policy Perspectives.* Washington, DC: National Academy Press, 1987.
3. *John Naisbitt's Trend Letter.* 1993.
4. *Guides to the Evaluation of Permanent Impairment.* 4th ed. Chicago: American Medical Association; 1993.
5. *Report of the Commission on the Evaluation of Pain.* Rockville, Md: US Department of Health and Human Services. Social Security Administration; 1987. SSA publication 64-031.
6. Vasudevan SV. The relationship between pain and disability: an overview of the problem. *J Disability.* 1991;2:44–53.
7. Robertson G. Deluge of cases swamps disability programs: weak economy is blamed as overburdened bureaucracy struggles with backlog, *Richmond Times-Dispatch.* September 27, 1993.
8. Black RG, Chapman CR. The SAD index for clinical assessment of pain. In: Bonica JJ, Albe-Fessard D, eds. *Advances in Pain Research and Therapy.* Vol 1. New York: Raven Press; 1975: 301–305.
9. Turk DC, Rudy TE. The robustness of an empirically derived taxonomy of chronic pain patients. *Pain.* 1990;43:27–35.
10. Keefe FJ, Block AR. Development of an observation method for assessing pain behavior in chronic low back patients. *Behav Ther.* 1982;13:363–375.
11. Fisher AG. *Assessment of Motor and Process Skills Manual* [unpublished test manual]. Research ed. 7.0. Fort Collins, Colo: Colorado State University; 1994.
12. Marcus N, Chair, Committee to Establish Uniform Outcome Measures for Pain Treatment Programs. *Conference Report.* Washington, DC: American Academy of Pain Medicine; 1994.
13. Price DD, McGrath PA, Rafii A, Buckingham B. The validation of visual analogue scales as ratio scale measures for chronic and experimental pain. *Pain.* 1993;17:45–56.

14. Granger CV, Hamilton BB. The Uniform Data System for Medical Rehabilitation report of first admissions for 1992. *Am J Phys Med Rehabil.* 1994;73:51–55.

15. Hurri H. The Swedish back school in chronic low back pain II. *Scand J Rehabil Med.* 1989;21:41–44.

16. Gerhardt JJ. Measurements of ranges of motion and strength in evaluation of impairment. *J Disabil.* 1993;3:121–139.

17. Heinemann AW, Linacre JM, Wright BD, Hamilton BB, Granger C. Prediction of rehabilitation outcomes with disability measures. *Arch Phys Med Rehabil.* 1994;75:133–143.

18. Steig RL. The futility of physical testing in the assessment of disability. *APS J.* 1994;3:187–190.

19. Tait RC, Pollard CA, Margolis RB, Duckro PN, Krause SJ. The Pain Disability Index: psychometric and validity data. *Arch Phys Med Rehabil.* 1987;68:438–441.

20. Jensen MP, Karoly P, Braver S. The measurement of clinical pain intensity: a comparison of six methods. *Pain.* 1986;27:117–126.

21. Gracely RH. Evaluation of multidimensional pain scales. *Pain.* 1992;48:297–300.

22. Covington EC, Currie KO. Pain treatment program evaluation: science and sorcery. *APS Bull.* 1994;4:9–14.

23. *Moothart v Bowen,* 934 F2d 114 (7th Cir 1991).

24. *Dixon v Sullivan,* 83 CIV 7001 WCC (SD NY 1992).

25. Social Security Disability Benefits Reform Act of 1984, Pub L No. 98-460.

26. Merskey H. International Association for the Study of Pain classification of chronic pain: descriptions of chronic pain syndromes and definitions of pain terms. *Pain.* 1986;(suppl 3):S1–S225.

27. Chabal C, Jacobson L, Chaney E, Mariano AJ. Chronic nonmalignant pain: a syndrome not a diagnosis. *APS J.* 1994;3:138–139.

28. Melzak R. *Pain Measurement and Assessment.* New York: Raven Press; 1983.

29. Turk DC, Rudy TE. Toward an empirically derived taxonomy of chronic pain patients: integration of psychological assessment data. *J Consult Clin Psychol.* 1988;56:233–238.

30. Bergner M, Babbit RA, Pollard WE. The Sickness Impact Profile: reliability of a health status measure. *Med Care.* 1976;14:146–155.

31. McHorney C, Ware JE Jr, Racek AE. The MOS 36-item short-form health survey (SF-36), II: psychometric and clinical tests of validity in measuring physical and mental health constructs. *Med Care.* 1993;31:247–263.

32. McArthur DL, Cohen MJ, Schandler SL. Rasch analysis of functional assessment scales: an example using pain behaviors. *Arch Phys Med Rehabil.* 1991;72:296–304.

33. Derogatis LR. *SCL-90 Administration, Scoring and Procedures Manual.* Baltimore: Johns Hopkins University Press; 1977.

34. Boyd JH, Weissman MM, Thompson D, Myers JK. Screening for depression in a community sample: understanding the discrepancies between depression symptoms and diagnostic scales. *Arch Gen Psychiatry.* 1982;39:1195–1200.

35. Tait RC. Psychological factors in the assessment of disability among patients with chronic pain. *J Back Muscul Rehabil.* 1993; 3(1):20–44.

36. Turk DC, Helmes E. What types of useful information do the MMPI and MMPI-2 provide on patients with chronic pain? *APS Bull.* 1994;4:1–5.

37. Epstein NB, Baldwin LM, Bishop DS. The McMaster Family Assessment Device. *J Marital Fam Ther.* 1983;9:171–180.

38. Granger CV, Wright B. Looking ahead to the use of functional assessment in ambulatory physiatric and primary care. *Phys Med Rehabil Clin North Am.* 1993;4:1–11.

39. Waddell G, McCullock JA, Kummel E, Venner RM. Nonorganic physical signs in low-back pain. *Spine.* 1980;5:117–125.

40. Hall KM, Hamilton BB, Gorden WA, Zasler ND. Characteristics and comparisons of functional assessment indices: Disability Rating Scale, Functional Independence Measure, and Functional Assessment Measure. *J Head Trauma Rehabil.* 1993;8:60–74.

41. Granger CV, Gresham GE. New developments in functional assessment. *Phys Med Rehabil Clin North Am.* 1993;4:417–611.

42. Hammonds W, Brena SF. Pain classification and vocational evaluation in chronic pain states. In: Melzack R, ed. *Pain Measurement and Assessment.* New York: Raven Press, 1983:197–203.

43. Fishbain DA, Rosomoff HL, Goldberg M, et al. The prediction of return to the workplace after multi-disciplinary pain center treatment. *Clin J Pain.* 1993;9:3–15.

44. Richards JS, Nepomuceno C, Riles M, Suer Z. Assessing pain behavior: the UAB pain behavior scale. *Pain.* 1982;14:393–398.

45. Tearnan BH, Lewandowski MJ. The behavioral assessment of pain questionnaire: the development and validation of a comprehensive self-report instrument. *AJPM.* 1992;2:181–191.

46. Aronoff GM. *Pain Centers: A Revolution in Health Care.* New York: Raven Press; 1988.

47. Williams RC. Toward a set of reliable and valid measures for chronic pain assessment and outcome research. *Pain.* 1988;35:239–251.

48. Feuerstein M. More than meets the eye: It's not simply an image problem—challenges facing chronic pain management clinics. *APS Bull.* 1994;4:1–3, 18.

49. Martin T. High tech, high cost health care system. *Whole Earth Review.* 1993;Fall:68–73.

50. Holzman AD, Rudy TE, Gerber KE, et al. Chronic pain: a multiple-setting comparison of patient characteristics. *J Behav Med.* 1985;8:411–422.

51. Kolar E, Hartz A, Roumm A, Ryan L, Jones R, Kirchdoerfer E. Factors associated with severity of symptoms in patients with chronic unexplained muscular aching. *Ann Rheum Dis.* 1989;48: 317–321.

52. Moldofsky H. Nonrestorative sleep and symptoms after a febrile illness in patients with fibrositis and chronic fatigue syndromes. *J Rheumatol Suppl.* 1989;19:150–153.

53. Mellman Lazarus Lake, Inc. Presentation of Findings. Washington, DC: May Day Fund, 1993.

54. Committee on House Ways and Means, US House of Representatives. *Overview of Entitlement Programs (1993 Greenbook).* Washington, DC: US Government Printing Office; 1993.

55. Aronoff GM. Chronic pain and the disability epidemic. *Clin J Pain.* 1991;7:330–338.

56. Social Security Act 42 USC, §423. Amended by Social Security Disability Reform Act of 1984, Pub L No. 98-460.

57. SSA Reg 404.1508/416.908.

58. SSA Reg 404.1529/416-929.

59. *Carr v Sullivan,* 772 F Supp 522 (East Dist Wash 1991).

60. Graham C, Bond SS, Gerkousch MM, Cook MR. Use of the McGill Pain Questionnaire in the assessment of cancer pain: replicability and consistency. *Pain.* 1980;8:377–387.

61. Hunter M, Phillips C, Rachman S. Memory for pain. *Pain.* 1979;6: 35–46.

62. Crockett DJ, Parkachin KM, Craig KD. Factors of the language of pain in patient and normal volunteer groups. *Pain.* 1977;4:175–182.

63. Leavitt F, Garron DC, Whisler WW, Sheinkop MB. Affective and sensory dimensions of pain. *Pain.* 1977;4:273–281.

64. Priets EJ, Hopson L, Bradley LA, et al. The language of low back pain: factor structure of the McGill Pain Questionnaire. *Pain.* 1980;8:11–20.

65. Flor H, Turk DC, Rudy TE. Relationship of pain impact and significant other reinforcement of pain behaviors: the mediating role of gender, marital status and marital satisfaction. *Pain.* 1989;38: 45–50.

66. Turk DC, Kerns RD. Conceptual issues in the assessment of clinical pain. *Int J Psychiatry Med.* 1983;13:57–58.

67. Faucett JA, Levine JD. The contributions of interpersonal conflict to chronic pain in the presence or absence of organic pathology. *Pain.* 1991;44:35–43.

68. Meade TW, Dyer S, Browne W, Townsend J, Frank AO. Low back pain of mechanical origin: randomized comparison of chiropractic and hospital outpatient treatment. *Br Med J.* 1990;300:1431–1437.

69. Triano JJ, Schultz AB. Correlation of objective measure of trunk motion and muscle function with low-back disability ratings. *Spine.* 1987;12:561–565.

70. Olson DH, McCubbin HJ, Barnes H, Jarsen A, Muxen M, Wilson M. Family inventories [manual]. St. Paul, Minn: Family Social Science; 1982.

71. Orme JG, Reis J, Herz EJ. Factorial and discriminant validity of the Center for Epidemiological Studies Depression (CES-D) Scale. *J Clin Psychol.* 1986;42:28–33.

72. Aneshensel CS, Clark VA, Frerichs RR. Race, ethnicity, and depression: a confirmatory analysis. *J Pers Soc Psychol.* 1983;44: 385–398.

73. Ross CE, Mirowsky J. Components of depressed mood in married men and women: the Center for Epidemiologic Studies Depression Scale. *Am J Epidemiol.* 1984;119:997–1004.

74. Pain Assessment Instruments Development Project. *Results of the Intrarater and Interrater Reliability of Pain Instruments: Report to SSA.* Richmond, Va: Virginia Commonwealth University/Medical College of Virginia; 1992.

75. Pain Assessment Instruments Development Project. *Results of Construct Validity Tests: Report to SSA.* Richmond, Va: Virginia Commonwealth University/Medical College of Virginia; 1992.

76. Pain Assessment Instruments Development Project. *Results of Concurrent Validity Tests: Report to SSA.* Richmond, Va: Virginia Commonwealth University/Medical College of Virginia; 1992.

77. Flor H, Fydrich T, Turk DC. Efficacy of multidisciplinary pain treatment centers: a meta-analytic review. *Pain.* 1992; 49:221–230.

78. Conley S. Health-related disabilities, pain and employment: initial impact of The Americans with Disabilities Act of 1990. *J Vocat Rehabil.* 1995:106.

79. Elswick RK, Kisk CW. *Sample Size Calculations* [pamphlet]. Richmond, Va: Medical College of Virginia; 1988.

80. Fredrickson BE, Trief PM, Van Beveren P, Yuan HA, Baum G. Rehabilitation of the patient with chronic back pain: a search for outcome predictors. *Spine.* 1988;13:351–353.

81. Rossignol M, Suissa S, Abenhaim L. Working disability due to occupational back pain: three-year follow-up of 2,300 compensated workers in Quebec. *J Occup Med.* 1988;30:502–505.

82. Pain Assessment Instruments Development Project. *Results of Pilot Tests for All Pain Assessment Instruments: Report to SSA.* Richmond, Va: Virginia Commonwealth University/Medical College of Virginia; 1991.

83. Cohen J, Cohen P. *Applied Multiple Regression/Correlation Analysis for the Behavioral Sciences.* 2nd ed. Hillsdale, NJ: Erlbaum; 1983.

84. Morrison DF. *Multivariate Statistical Methods.* New York: McGraw-Hill; 1967.

85. Cerny BA, Kaiser HF. A study of a measure of sampling adequacy for factor-analytic correlation matrices. *Mult Behav Res.* 1977;12:43–47.

86. Pain Assessment Instruments Development Project. *Results of Content Validity Tests: Report to SSA.* Richmond, Va: Virginia Commonwealth University/Medical College of Virginia; 1993.

87. Malone MD, Strube MJ. Meta-analysis of non-medical treatments for chronic pain. *Pain.* 1988;34:231–244.

88. Cote JA, Buckley MR, Best RJ. Combining methodologies in the construct validation process: an empirical illustration. *J Psychol.* 1987;121:301–309.

89. Rucker KS, Metzler HM. Predicting subsequent employment status of SSA disability applicants with chronic pain. *Clin J Pain.* 1995;11:22–35.

Additional Reading

Ackerman MD, Stevens MJ. Acute and chronic pain: pain dimensions and psychological status. *J Clin Psychol.* 1989;45:223–228.

Beck AT, Beck RW. Screening depressed patients in family practice: a rapid technic. *Postgrad Med.* 1972;52:81–85.

Blumer D, Heilbronn M. Chronic pain as a variant of depressive disease: the pain-prone disorder. *J Nerv Ment Dis.* 1982;170:381–406.

Chapman CR, Bonica JJ. Chronic pain. *Curr Concepts.* 1985;August: 1–68.

Davidson J, Krishnan R, France R, Pelton S. Neurovegetative symptoms in chronic pain and depression. *J Affect Dis.* 1985;9:213–218.

Engel GL. "Psychogenic" pain and the pain-prone patient. *Am J Med.* 1959;26:899–918.

Fields H, ed. *Pain.* New York, McGraw-Hill; 1987.

Flor H, Turk DC, Rudy TE. Relationship of pain impact and significant other reinforcement of pain behaviors: the mediating role of gender, marital status and marital satisfaction. *Pain.* 1989;38:45–50.

Fordyce W. *Behavioral methods for chronic pain and illness.* St. Louis: Mosby; 1976.

Kamerow DB, Pincus HA, MacDonald DI. Alcohol abuse, other drug abuse, and mental disorders in medical practice: prevalence, costs, recognition, and treatment. *JAMA.* 1986;255:2054–2057.

Maruta T, Swanson DW, Finlayson RE. Drug abuse and dependency in patients with chronic pain. *Mayo Clin Proc* 1979;54:241–244.

Melzack R, Casey KL. Sensory motivational and central control of determinants of pain. In: Kenshalo DR, ed. *The Skin Senses.* Springfield, Ill: Charles C Thomas; 1968:423–439.

Mohamed SN, Weisz GM, Waring EM. The relationship of chronic pain to depression, marital adjustment, and family dynamics. *Pain.* 1978;5:285–292.

National Council of Disability Determination Directors Report. Rockville, MD: NCDDD; 1993.

Pelz M, Merskey H. A description of the psychological effects of chronic painful lesions. *Pain.* 1982;14:293–301.

Report of the Commission on the Evaluation of Pain. Rockville, Md: US Department of Health and Human Services. Social Security Administration; 1987. SSA publication 64-031.

Romano JM, Turner JA. Chronic pain and depression: does the evidence support a relationship? *Psychol Bull.* 1985;97:18–34.

Stimmel B. *Pain, Analgesia, and Addiction: The Pharmacologic Treatment of Pain.* New York: Raven Press; 1983.

Thompson SC. Will it hurt less if I can control it? A complex answer to a simple question. *Psychol Bull.* 1981;90:89–101.

Turk DC, Kerns RD. Conceptual issues in the assessment of clinical pain. *Int J Psychiatry Med.* 1983;13:1983–1984.

Glossary of Abbreviations

ADA Americans with Disabilities Act

ADL Activities of daily living

ALJ Administrative law judge

ANOVA Analysis of variance

CSPI Patient instrument from the Pain Assessment Instrument

CSPI-SO Patient instrument for significant others from the Pain Assessment Instrument

FCE Functional capacity evaluation

FIM Functional independence measure

IPR Integrated Pain Report from the Pain Assessment Instrument

MMPAP Multidimensional Multiperspective Pain Assessment Protocol

MTMM Multitrait-multimethod analysis

PAI Pain Assessment Instrument

PAID Pain Assessment Instrument Development Project. Research contract awarded to Virginia Commonwealth University, June 1990. Principal investigator, KS Rucker, M.D.

PSI Pain Screening Instrument from the Pain Assessment Instrument

PSPI-CP The consulting physician form from the Pain Assessment Instrument

PSPI-TP The treating physician form from the Pain Assessment Instrument

ROM Range of motion

SNK Student-Newman-Keuls post hoc means tests

SSA Social Security Administration

SSDI Social Security Disability Insurance—disabled workers' entitlement program

VAS Visual analogue scale

1 | Pain Screening Instrument

PAIN ASSESSMENT INSTRUMENT

Patient's Name: _____
                          Last   First   Middle Initial

Social Security Number: _ _ _-_ _-_ _ _ _   Today's Date: _ _/_ _/_ _

Do you have pain related to the condition for which you are applying for disability?
___Yes ___ No

If **No**, you are finished with this form. If **Yes**, please continue.

This form will help us learn more about your pain and how it affects your life. You know your pain better than anyone else. Please read and answer each question carefully. Give only one answer per question.

1. When did your pain begin? _ _/_ _
                                                  Month/Year

2. In the **past six months** how often have you had pain? ___
      1 = Less than once a month   4 = At least once a day
      2 = At least once a month   5 = Several times per day to continuously
      3 = At least once a week

3. In the **past six months**, when you have had pain, how long has the pain usually lasted? ___
      1 = 5 minutes or less   4 = Over 1 day to 1 week
      2 = Over 1 hour to 1 day   5 = Over 1 week to continuously
      3 = Over 1 hour to 1 day

4. What was the usual intensity of your pain in the past week? ___
      1 = None to minimal   4 = Strong
      2 = Mild   5 = Extreme
      3 = Moderate

5. Please check in the columns the amount of unpleasantness your pain has caused you at the usual level and at the highest level:

Level	1 = Neutral	2 = Unpleasant	3 = Very Unpleasant	4 = Distressing	5 = Unbearable
a. Usual intensity in the past week					
b. Highest intensity in the past week					

6. In the past week, how often have you felt that

	1 = Always	2 = Most times	3 = Often	4 = Sometimes	5 = Never
a. your situation is hopeless?					
b. you will never be able to work again?					
c. you will never be able to do things you used to enjoy?					

APPENDIX

2 | Patient Assessment

PAIN ASSESSMENT INSTRUMENT

Completed by: _____

PATIENT ASSESSMENT

Patient's Name: _____

Last   First   Middle Initial

Social Security Number: _ _ _-_ _-_ _ _ _   Today's Date: _ _/_ _/_ _

Instructions
You know your pain better than anyone else does. These forms will help us learn more about your pain and how it affects your life. Read each question carefully, and either check or write the number of the best answer in the blank. Please give only one answer per question.

Start Time: _____ A.M./P.M.

I. Pain Descriptions and Background Information

1. Is pain your primary health problem? _____ Yes _____ No

If **No**, what is your primary health problem? _____

2. What is your current weight? _____ lb

3. What is your height? _____ inches

4. Are you right handed or left handed? _____

1 = Right

2 = Left

3 = Both the same

Please show your pain on this diagram:

```
┌─────────────────────────────────────┐
│                                      │
│                                      │
│                                      │
│                                      │
│                                      │
│                                      │
│                                      │
│                                      │
│                                      │
│                                      │
│                                      │
│                                      │
│                                      │
│                                      │
│                                      │
└─────────────────────────────────────┘
```

5. Onset Date of Pain: _ _/_ _
                         Month/Year

    History of Pain: _____
    _____
    _____
    _____

6. Does the pain radiate to other areas? _____
    1 = Yes   2 = No

7. Is the pain a small point or a large area? ___
    1 = Point   2 = Area

8. Is the pain on the surface or deep? ___
    1 = Surface   2 = Deep

9. In the past 6 months how often have you had pain? ___
    1 = Less than once a month   4 = At least once a day
    2 = At least once a month   5 = Several times per day to continuously
    3 = At least once a week

10. If you have had pain-free periods in the past 6 months, how long do they usually last? ___

    0 = No pain-free periods   3 = Days
    1 = Minutes   4 = Weeks
    2 = Hours   5 = Months

11. In the past 6 months, when you have had pain, how long has the pain usually lasted? ___

    1 = 5 minutes or less   4 = More than 1 day to 1 week
    2 = More than 5 minutes to 1 hour   5 = More than 1 week to continuously
    3 = More than 1 hour to 1 day

12. In the past 6 months, what time of day has your pain been the worst? ___

    1 = Always the same level of severity
    2 = When you first get up
    3 = Morning
    4 = Afternoon
    5 = Evening
    6 = Right before bedtime
    7 = At night, when you are trying to sleep
    8 = Gets worse and better, but no specific pattern
    9 = Both morning and evening

13. In the past 6 months

    a. How many different doctors have you seen for pain? ___
    b. How many times have you seen a doctor or health specialist for pain? ___
    c. How many emergency room visits have you had for pain? ___
    d. How many hospitalizations have you had for pain? ___
    e. How many days were you in the hospital for pain? ___

14. In the **past 6 months**, how often has the pain made it hard to get to sleep? ___

    1 = Not at all   4 = Almost every night
    2 = Some nights   5 = Every night
    3 = Most nights

15. In the **past 6 months**, how often has the pain awakened you from sleep? ___

    1 = Not at all   4 = Almost every night
    2 = Some nights   5 = Every night
    3 = Most nights

16. How difficult is it to put up with or cope with your pain? ___

    1 = Easy   4 = Very difficult
    2 = Inconvenient   5 = Almost impossible
    3 = Troublesome

17. How much does the pain interfere with what you want to do? ___

    1 = No restrictions   4 = A great barrier

    2 = Minor interference   5 = Hinders all activities

    3 = Moderate obstacle

18. Have you ever resigned from a job without another job to go to? ___ Yes ___ No

    If **yes**, how many times? ___

There are two parts of pain that we are interested in assessing:

    1. The **intensity** of the painful sensation

    2. How **unpleasant** or disturbing it is to have the pain

The difference between these two parts of pain may be made clearer if you think of listening to a sound, such as a sound coming from a radio. As the volume of the sound increases, you can be asked how loud it sounds or how unpleasant it is to you. The **intensity** of painful sensation is like loudness; the **unpleasantness** of pain depends on the intensity and on **what it means to you**. Although some pains may be equally intense and unpleasant, we would like you to rate these two parts of pain separately.

19. Indicate the **intensity of painful sensation** when your pain was at the following levels:

Level	1 = None to Minimal	2 = Mild	3 = Moderate	4 = Strong	5 = Extreme
a. Right now					
b. Lowest intensity in the past week					
c. Usual intensity in the past week					
d. Highest intensity in the past week					

20. Indicate the amount of unpleasantness your pain has caused you when your pain was at the following levels:

Level	1 = Neutral	2 = Unpleasant	3 = Very Unpleasant	4 = Distressing	5 = Unbearable
a. Right now					
b. Lowest intensity in the past week					
c. Usual intensity in the past week					
d. Highest intensity in the past week					

21. In the past 6 months, how often

	1 = Always	2 = Most times	3 = Often	4 = Sometimes	5 = Never
a. have you found yourself talking about your pain?					
b. do you brace yourself or shift positions when standing or sitting because of pain?					
c. has your significant other been supportive or helpful when you are in pain?					
d. have you been able to predict when your pain will start, get better, or get worse?					
e. have you had sexual difficulties?					
f. have you had problems remembering your next task?					
g. have you had fights or disagreements with your significant other?					
h. have you had disagreements with or avoided other family members?					
i. have you felt self-confident?					
j. have you felt good about others?					
k. have you worked in your yard or garden?					

22. Please check in the columns below how much each of the following activities or conditions causes pain. Do not include unusual or prolonged activity.

Activity	1 = Not at All	2 = Very Little	3 = Moderate	4 = A Lot
a. Standing				
b. Walking				
c. Sitting				
d. Lifting/carrying				
e. Pushing/pulling				
f. Climbing stairs				
g. Bending/stooping/kneeling				
h. Reaching				
i. Handling/feeling/using fingers				
j. Talking/listening				
k. Reading/watching TV				
l. Extreme cold				
m. Extreme heat				

Activity	1 = Not at All	2 = Very Little	3 = Moderate	4 = A Lot
n. Temperature change				
o. Noise/vibration				
p. Exposure to fumes/odors/gases				
q. High speed work (fast assembly or meeting deadlines)				

23. Please check in the columns how much each of the following activities or conditions affects you **when you are in pain**:

Activity	1 = Pain Better	2 = No Change	3 = Pain Worse	4 = Pain Much Worse
a. Standing				
b. Walking				
c. Sitting				
d. Lifting/carrying				
e. Pushing/pulling				
f. Climbing stairs				
g. Bending/stooping/kneeling				
h. Reaching				
i. Handling/feeling/using fingers				
j. Talking/listening				
k. Reading/watching TV				
l. Extreme cold				
m. Extreme heat				
n. Temperature change				
o. Noise/vibration				
p. Exposure to fumes/odors/gases				
q. High speed work (fast assembly or meeting deadlines)				

24. How does your significant other respond to you when you are in pain?

Response	1 = Always	2 = Most times	3 = Often	4 = Sometimes	5 = Never
a. Helps me with my job or duties					
b. Asks what he/she can do to help					
c. Gets irritated with me					
d. Gets frustrated with me					
e. Gets me something to eat or drink					

25. In the **past week**, how often have you felt that

	1 = Always	2 = Most Times	3 = Often	4 = Sometimes	5 = Never
a. you will always have health problems?					
b. your situation is hopeless?					
c. you will never be able to work again?					
d. you will never be able to do things you used to enjoy?					
e. you have no motivation to get better?					

26. In the **past 6 months**, how frequently has the pain limited your ability to

	1 = Always	2 = Most Times	3 = Often	4 = Sometimes	5 = Never
a. concentrate?					
b. understand instructions?					
c. communicate with others?					
d. take care of your personal needs (dressing, grooming, bathing, etc.)?					
e. move throughout your home (up and down stairs, inside and outside, etc.)?					
f. complete housecleaning and household tasks (washing dishes, scrubbing floors, etc.)?					
g. use your hands to do fine work (sewing, writing, using screwdriver, etc.)?					
h. get to places outside of walking distance by driving, taking the bus, or other means?					
i. tolerate minor irritations that would not normally make you angry?					

27. How many, if any, cigarettes do you smoke each day? ___

1 = Don't smoke   4 = 21 to 40 per day
2 = Less than 5 per day   5 = More than 40 per day
3 = 5 to 20 per day

28. How often do you drink alcohol? ___

1 = Never   4 = Frequently (several times a week)
2 = Rarely (less than once a week)   5 = Daily
3 = Socially (once a week)

If you drink alcohol

28a. Have you ever had a period of self imposed abstinence? ___ Yes ___ No
28b. Does your significant other get upset when you drink? ___ Yes ___ No

28c. Has anyone ever annoyed you by criticizing your drinking? ___ Yes ___ No

28d. Do you sometimes drink in the morning to steady your nerves or get rid of a hangover? ___ Yes ___ No

28e. Do you ever drink to lessen the pain? ___ Yes ___ No

29. How often do you use recreational drugs (drugs used but not for a medical problem)? ___

    1 = Never   4 = Frequently (several per week)
    2 = Rarely (less than once a week)   5 = Daily
    3 = Socially (once a week)

30. Have you ever been hospitalized for emotional problems related to your pain?
    ___ Yes ___ No

31. Have you been seen by a mental health specialist (psychiatrist, psychologist, professional counselor) for treatment of this pain (not a one-time evaluation)?
    ___ Yes ___ No

    If the answer to question 31 is **yes**,

    31a. How many times have you seen the mental health specialist? ___

    31b. Did the consultation help? ___ Yes ___ No

    Please explain:_____
    _____
    _____

32. Do you ever need medication for pain? ___ Yes ___ No

33. Have you ever taken medication for pain in the past 6 months? ___ Yes ___ No
    If the answer to question 33 is **yes**, please answer the following questions concerning your medications.

    33a. How often do you take medicine for your pain? ___

    1 = Less than once a week   4 = Three to four times a day
    2 = Several times a week   5 = Five or more times a day
    3 = One or two times a day

    33b. Have you needed more pain medications in the past 6 months than your doctor prescribed? ___ Yes ___ No

    33c. How likely is it that you will always need medication for pain? ___

    1 = Definitely   4 = Unlikely
    2 = Likely   5 = Extremely unlikely
    3 = Possibly

    33d. On the average, do the medicines you take ___

    1 = always take the pain away   4 = usually make the pain less
    2 = always make the pain less   5 = provide little or no relief
    3 = usually takes the pain away

33e. On the average, how long do the medicines provide relief? ___

1 = Not at all   4 = 3 to less than 6 hours

2 = Less than 1 hour   5 = More than 6 hours

3 = 1 hour to less than 3 hours

34. In the **past 6 months**, how frequently and severely did you feel

	Frequency			Severity		
	0 = Never	1 = Sometimes	2 = Often	1 = Mildly	2 = Moderate	3 = Severely
a. depressed						
b. frustrated						
c. anxious						
d. angry						
e. guilty						

II. Historical Information

Please try to remember back before you had the pain. To help us understand how your life has changed, we are going to ask several questions twice:

Before the pain, how often did you
In the past 6 months, how often did you

		1 = Always	2 = Most Times	3 = Often	4 = Sometimes	5 = Never
1. have problems completing jobs on time?	Before pain					
	Past 6 mo					
2. eat more or less than you should?	Before pain					
	Past 6 mo					
3. turn down social invitations such as community activities?	Before pain					
	Past 6 mo					
4. have disagreements or problems working with others?	Before pain					
	Past 6 mo					
5. go shopping (to the grocery store, department store, etc.)	Before pain					
	Past 6 mo					
6. exercise or stay fit (bicycling, walking, swimming, jogging)?	Before pain					
	Past 6 mo					
7. go to restaurants?	Before pain					
	Past 6 mo					
8. do your laundry (at home or at a Laundromat)?	Before pain					
	Past 6 mo					
9. drive when traveling by car?	Before pain					
	Past 6 mo					

		1 = Always	2 = Most Times	3 = Often	4 = Sometimes	5 = Never
10. prepare and cook complete meals?	Before pain					
	Past 6 mo					
11. attend or participate in recreational activities outside your home (go to movies, the park, bowling, etc.)?	Before pain					
	Past 6 mo					

III. Medical Information

1. Have you had any of the following tests or treatments for this problem?

Procedure	Yes	No
a. Surgical procedures		
b. Nerve blocks		
c. Chiropractic care		
d. Traction		
e. Shots, injections		
f. Acupuncture		
g. Electromyogram (EMG)		
h. Myelogram		
i. Physical therapy		
j. Other (specify)		

2. Please indicate in the appropriate box the **number of family members** who have had the following medical problems. Count yourself as 1. When referring to spouse, please include current spouse only.

Medical Problem	You	Spouse	Parent or Child	Grand-parent	Brother or Sister
a. Headache					
b. Stroke					
c. Arthritis					
d. Chronic pain					
e. Brain tumor					
f. Cancer					
g. High blood pressure					
h. Epilepsy					
i. Heart attack					
j. Angina					
k. Ulcer (duodenum, stomach)					
l. Thyroid disease					

IV. Functional Abilities and Restrictions

1. If your pain were reduced to an acceptable level, list the things you would do that your current pain level keeps you from doing. Be specific.

    a. _____

    b. _____

    c. _____

2. How many times in a row can you do the following activities (before your pain causes you to stop?

Activity	Not at all	1–4	5–9	10–19	20–39	40 or more
a. Reach overhead						
b. Bend, squat or stoop						

3. Which of the following items can you lift from the floor to a counter (your waist level)?

Item	1 = Easily	2 = With Mild Pain	3 = With Moderate Pain	4 = With Severe Pain	5 = Not at All
a. Pencil, candy, or paper					
b. 5-lb bag of rice, flour, sugar					
c. 12-pack of canned drinks					
d. Case of canned drinks					

The following questions are groups of statements. Please read all statements in each group, then pick out the one statement in that group which best describes the way you fool today, *right now*!! Be sure to read all statements in each group before making your choice.

Group A ___
3 = I am so sad or unhappy that I can't stand it.
2 = I am blue or sad all the time, and I can't snap out of it.
1 = I feel sad or blue.
0 = I do not feel sad.

Group B ___
3 = I feel that the future is hopeless and that things cannot improve.
2 = I feel I have nothing to look forward to.
1 = I feel discouraged about the future.
0 = I am not particularly pessimistic or discouraged about the future.

Group C ___
3 = I feel I am a complete failure as a person (parent, husband, wife).
2 = As I look back on my life, all I can see is a lot of failures.
1 = I feel I have failed more than the average person has.
0 = I do not feel like a failure.

133

Group D ___
3 = I am dissatisfied with everything.
2 = I don't get satisfaction out of anything anymore.
1 = I don't enjoy things the way I used to.
0 = I am not particularly dissatisfied.

Group E ___
3 = I feel as though I am very bad or worthless.
2 = I feel quite guilty.
1 = I feel bad or unworthy a good part of the time.
0 = I don't feel particularly guilty.

Group F ___
3 = I hate myself.
2 = I am disgusted with myself.
1 = I am disappointed in myself.
0 = I don't feel disappointed in myself.

Group G ___
3 = I would kill myself if I had the chance.
2 = I have definite plans about committing suicide.
1 = I feel I would be better off dead.
0 = I don't have any thoughts of harming myself.

Group H ___
3 = I have lost all of my interest in other people and don't care about them at all.
2 = I have lost most of my interest in other people and have little feeling for them.
1 = I am less interested in other people than I used to be.
0 = I have not lost interest in other people.

Group I ___
3 = I can't make any decisions at all anymore.
2 = I have great difficulty in making decisions.
1 = I try to put off making decisions.
0 = I make decisions about as well as ever.

Group J ___
3 = I feel that I am ugly or repulsive looking.
2 = I feel that there are permanent changes in my appearance, and they make me look unattractive.
1 = I am worried that I am looking old or unattractive.
0 = I don't feel that I look any worse than I used to.

Group K ___
3 = I can't do any work at all.
2 = I have to push myself very hard to do anything.
1 = It takes extra effort to get started at doing something.
0 = I can work about as well as before.

Group L ___
3 = I get too tired to do anything.
2 = I get tired from doing anything.
1 = I get tired more easily than I used to.
0 = I don't get any more tired than usual.

Group M ___
3 = I have no appetite at all anymore.
2 = My appetite is much worse now.
1 = My appetite is not as good as it used to be.
0 = My appetite is no worse than usual.

Ending time: _____ A.M./P.M.

APPENDIX

3 | Physician Assessment

PAIN ASSESSMENT INSTRUMENT

Patient's Name: _____   SSN: _ _ _-_ _-_ _ _ _
Physician's Name: _____   Date of Exam: _ _/_ _/_ _
Clinic: _____

Start Time: _____ A.M./P.M.

1. How many years have you or did you treat this patient? ___
   Less than 1   1   2   3   4   5   6   7   8   9   10   11–20   More than 20

2. How many times have you examined this patient (before today)? ___
   0   1   2   3   4   5   6   7   8   9   10   11–20   More than 20

3. Have you previously treated the patient for unrelated injuries? ___ Yes ___ No

I. Description and Onset of Present Impairment
4. Onset event: Pain began with or is caused by which of the following? ___

   1 = Trauma   9 = Surgery
   2 = Infection   10 = Stress, physical or emotional
   3 = Neoplasm   11 = Perinatal factor
   4 = Congenital: birth defect or deformity 12 = Vascular
   5 = Psychological/psychogenic   13 = Unknown
   6 = Degenerative   14 = Unspecified
   7 = Demyelinative/neurogenic   15 = Overuse/repetitive/microtrauma
   8 = Toxic metabolic

5. Is pain the patient's chief complaint? ___ Yes ___ No

6. Please indicate the primary diagnosis of the patient's pain or impairment causing the pain and up to two other diagnoses in the order of importance. Please list the ICD-9 code if known.

   1. _____
   2. _____
   3. _____

137

7. On the basis of your examination, estimate how often the patient's pain occurs.

   a. Baseline ___   b. Flare up ___

   1 = Less often than once a month   4 = At least once a day
   2 = At least once a month   5 = Several times per day to continuously
   3 = At least once a week

8. In your opinion and on the basis of your examination, how intense is the patient's usual pain? ___

   1 = None to minimal   4 = Strong
   2 = Mild   5 = Extreme
   3 = Moderate

9. Check *Yes* or *No* for each of the following types of medications if the patient is currently taking it to relieve pain or to alleviate the underlying condition.

   a. Antiinflammatory ___ Yes ___ No
   b. Narcotic analgesic ___ Yes ___ No
   c. Nonnarcotic analgesic (e.g., acetaminophen) ___ Yes ___ No
   d. Sedative/tranquilizer ___ Yes ___ No
   e. Tricyclic antidepressant ___ Yes ___ No
   f. Muscle relaxant, major (diazepam, baclofen) ___ Yes ___ No
   g. Muscle relaxant, minor (cyclobenzaprine) ___ Yes ___ No
   h. Anticonvulsant ___ Yes ___ No

10. Check *Yes* or *No* for each of these types of medications if they have previously been prescribed but subsequently discontinued to relieve the patient's pain or to alleviate the underlying condition.

   a. Antiinflammatory ___ Yes ___ No
   b. Narcotic analgesic ___ Yes ___ No
   c. Nonnarcotic analgesic (e.g., acetaminophen) ___ Yes ___ No
   d. Sedative/tranquilizer ___ Yes ___ No
   e. Tricyclic antidepressant ___ Yes ___ No
   f. Muscle relaxant, major (diazepam, baclofen) ___ Yes ___ No
   g. Muscle relaxant, minor (cyclobenzaprine) ___ Yes ___ No
   h. Anticonvulsant ___ Yes ___ No

11. Has the patient reported sleep disturbances? ___ Yes ___ No

12. Have you ever referred the patient to a mental health specialist for reasons other than a general evaluation? ___ Yes ___ No

   12a. If the answer to question 12 is **No**, do you think a referral is now indicated?
        ___ Yes ___ No

13. Has the patient been seen by a mental health specialist for reasons other than general evaluation? ___ Yes ___ No

14. How effective have the following treatments been? Also check whether the treatment provided temporary relief or long-term relief. If the treatment was not performed, no further answer is needed.

Treatment	0 = Not Performed	1 = Worse	2 = Moderate	3 = Marked	1 = Temporary (<2 wk)	2 = Long Term (>2 wk)
a. Surgery						
b. Nerve blocks						
c. Heat/cold						
d. Braces/casts/corsets						
e. Chiropractic/manipulation						
f. Exercise program						
g. TENS						
h. Traction						
i. Trigger point injections						
j. Acupuncture						
k. Massage/soft tissue mobilization						
l. Biofeedback/hypnosis/ relaxation						
m. Other: _____						

Please perform each of the following tests during the physical exam. Indicate the level of abnormality detected. *IE* = Insufficient evidence.

Test	Level of Abnormality					
	1 = None	2 = Slight	3 = Moderate	4 = Marked	5 = Extreme or Rigid	6 = IE
15. Abnormalities in range of motion						
a. Neck						
b. Low back						
c. Upper extremity: Right						
c. Upper extremity: Left						
d. Lower extremity: Right						
d. Lower extremity: Left						
16. Dysesthesia: Unpleasant and abnormal sensation; either spontaneous or evoked						
17. Hyperpathia: Increased reaction to a stimulus, especially a repetitive stimulus, and an increased threshold						

Test	Level of Abnormality					
	1 = None	2 = Slight	3 = Moderate	4 = Marked	5 = Extreme or Rigid	6 = IE
18. Autonomic dysfunction (e.g., cold extremity, tropic changes)						
19. Gait abnormalities						
20. Muscle atrophy						
21. Joint deformity						
22. Vascular abnormalities (pulse, blood pressure, edema, cyanosis, bruit, etc.)						
23. Muscle spasm (palpable and sustained taut band of muscles)						
24. Tenderness to palpation						
a. Radiates (trigger points)						
b. Does not radiate (tender points)						

25. In general, were the results of the neurologic examination normal? ___

    1 = Normal
    2 = Abnormal, related to pain complaint
    3 = Abnormal, unrelated to pain complaint
    4 = Not physiologic

26. How much support do laboratory studies give to the patient's complaints?

Study	Not Performed	Official Result Not Available	1 = No Support	2 = Mild Support	3 = Moderate Support	4 = Strong Support	5 = Unequivocal Support
a. Radiographs							
b. CT							
c. MRI							
d. Bone scan							
e. Electrodiagnostics							
f. Blood-studies							
g. Urine studies							
h. Other: _____							

II. Functional Abilities Estimation

When answering this section, please refer to the following criteria:

Never Patient prohibited from performing activity.
Rarely Less than 1 hour per day safe maximum effort.

Occasionally 1 to 3 hours per day safe maximum effort.

Frequently 4 to 5 hours per day safe maximum effort.

Continuously 6 to 8 hours per day safe maximum effort.

Sedentary work Lifting 10 pounds maximum and occasionally lifting and/or carrying articles such as dockers, ledgers or small tools. Although a sedentary job is defined as one that involves sitting, a certain amount of walking and standing often is necessary in carrying out job duties. Jobs are sedentary if walking and standing are required occasionally and all other sedentary criteria are met.

Light work Lifting 20 pounds or more maximum with frequent lifting and/or carrying objects weighing up to 10 pounds. Even though the weight lifted may be only a negligible amount, a job is in this category (1) when it requires walking or standing to a significant degree; or (2) when it requires sitting most of the time but entails pushing and pulling of arm and/or leg controls.

Medium work Lifting 50 pounds maximum with frequent lifting and/or carrying objects weighing up to 25 pounds.

Heavy work Lifting 100 pounds maximum with frequently lifting and/or carrying of objects weighing up to 50 pounds.

Sit/Stand Alternating work posture between sitting and standing.

Stand/Walk Alternating work posture between standing and walking.

On the basis of the entire exam, please provide your assessment of the patient's ability to perform the following activities:

1. How many hours (in an 8-hour day) can the patient be expected to perform the following types of work?

Type of Work	1 = Never	2 = Rarely (<1h)	3 = Occasionally (1–3 h)	4 = Frequently (4–5 h)	5 = Continuously (6–8 h)
a. Sedentary work					
b. Light work					
c. Medium work					
d. Heavy work					

2. In your estimation, how long can the patient perform the following activities continuously without break or interruption?

Activity	Not at All	<15 min	15–29 min	30–44 min	45–59 min	≥60 min
a. Sit						
b. Stand						

3. Are there medical restrictions on the patient's ability to perform work under any of the following conditions? (Check *Yes* or *No* for each option)

    a. Heat ___ Yes ___ No

    b. Cold ___ Yes ___ No

    c. Temperature changes ___ Yes ___ No

    e. Exposure to fumes/dust ___ Yes ___ No

    d. High speed working ___ Yes ___ No

4. What is the maximum weight (in pounds) the patient can lift in each of the following categories? (When responding, consider *occasionally* as approximately three times per hour, *repetitively* as approximately 20 times per hour, *counter* as a standard 36-inch height, and *overhead* as approximately 150 degrees' shoulder flexion.)

Lift	<1 lb	1–5 lb	6–25 lb	26–50 lb	>50 lb
a. Floor to counter occasionally					
b. Floor to counter repetitively					
c. Counter to counter occasionally					
d. Counter to counter repetitively					
e. Counter to overhead occasionally					
f. Counter to overhead repetitively					

5. How many hours (in an 8-hour day) can the patient be expected to perform the following activities?

Activity	1 = Never	2 = Rarely (<1 h)	3 = Occasionally (1–3 h)	4 = Frequently (4–5 h)	5 = Continuously (6–8 h)
a. Walk					
b. Sit					
c. Stand					
d. Lift (20 lb maximum with frequent repetitions)					
e. Push					
f. Pull					
g. Sit/stand					
h. Stand/walk					
i. Bend/stoop					
j. Climb					
k. Squat/kneel					
l. Simple grasping					
m. Fine hand and finger manipulations					
n. Sustained work requiring reaching overhead (shoulder flexion 150 degrees)					

6. In your estimation, how many times in a row can the patient perform the following activities to exhaustion or until pain forces the patient to stop?

Activity	None	1–4 Times	5–9 Times	10–19 Times	20–39 Times	40 or More
a. Reach overhead						
b. Squat or kneel						

7. Has the patient reached maximum medical improvement? ___ Yes ___ No

    7a. If the answer to question 7 is **No**, when can maximum improvement be expected? _____

        1 = Within the next 6 months from today's date

        2 = More than 6 months after today's date

8. In your estimation, what level of effort will the patient expend if a functional capacity evaluation is performed?

    1 = No effort   4 = Maximum effort

    2 = Minimal effort   5 = Extreme effort

    3 = Moderate effort

III. Social Functioning and Development

Please respond to the following questions on the basis of your perceptions about and interactions with the patient. **Do not ask the patient to provide this information.**

IE = Insufficient evidence

To what degree has the patient

	1 = None	2 = Slight	3 = Moderate	4 = Marked	5 = Extreme	6 = IE
1. displayed pain behavior signs (e.g., grimacing, shifting, audible indications)?						
2. talked about pain?						
3. displayed abnormal posturing or abnormal movement due to pain?						
4. experienced sleep disturbances due to pain?						
5. been inactive or sedentary because of pain?						
6. displayed frustration or anger due to pain?						
7. been sad or depressed because of pain?						
8. displayed nervousness or anxiety due to pain?						
9. exhibited more mood alterations than other patients with similar problems?						
10. used health care services compared with patients with similar problems?						
11. been compliant with prescribed care?						

	1 = None	2 = Slight	3 = Moderate	4 = Marked	5 = Extreme	6 = IE
12. expressed desire to undergo repeated painful diagnostic procedures or surgery?						

To what degree has the pain caused the patient to have difficulty with

	1 = None	2 = Slight	3 = Moderate	4 = Marked	5 = Extreme	6 = IE
13. light household tasks (e.g., dusting, cooking)?						
14. heavy household tasks (e.g., carrying wash, yard work)?						
15. light leisure activities (e.g., reading, watching TV)?						
16. exercising or staying fit (e.g., bicycling, walking, swimming, jogging)?						
17. participating in recreational activities outside the home (e.g., go to parks, movies, bowling)?						
18. moving about the house (e.g., up and down stairs, inside and outside)?						
19. traveling independently about town?						
20. performing personal hygiene, dressing and undressing independently?						
21. using hands to write letters, pay bills, etc?						
22. understanding and remembering complex instructions?						
23. completing tasks without help from spouse or others (e.g., recounting history of problem)?						
24. thinking clearly without impaired judgment?						
25. maintaining a relationship with a spouse or significant other?						
26. maintaining interpersonal relationships?						

IV. Physician's Assessment of Rehabilitation Potential

1. Which of the following definitions best describe the patient's pain situation? _____

   1 = Patient does not have chronic pain.
   2 = Chronic pain, inability to cope; insufficient documented impairment.
   3 = Chronic pain, competent coping; insufficient documented impairment.
   4 = Chronic pain, inability to cope; documented impairment sufficient.
   5 = Chronic pain, competent coping; documented impairment sufficient.

2. Did the patient react appropriately to the exam, or did the pain behaviors appear exaggerated? ___

   1 = Appropriate response   2 = Exaggerated response

3. In your estimation, how supportive is the patient's social support network (e.g., significant other, family, friends) in terms of providing emotional support and practical assistance that will enable the patient to effectively cope with the pain? (e.g., significant other, family, friends) ___

   1 = Very supportive   4 = Somewhat critical or unsympathetic
   2 = Somewhat supportive   5 = Intolerant
   3 = Ambivalent

4. If this patient were to have a sufficient support system (e.g., a very supportive family or significant other), how good a candidate do you believe he/she would be for participation in a rehabilitation program? ___

   1 = Excellent   4 = Poor
   2 = Good   5 = Definitely not a candidate
   3 = Average   6 = Does not need

5. How motivated do you believe this patient has been or would be in terms of changing his or her lifestyle (e.g., take lower pay, move, take a less desirable job) to be rehabilitated? ___

   1 = Extremely motivated   4 = Slightly motivated
   2 = Moderately motivated   5 = Not motivated
   3 = Somewhat motivated

6. To what extent are the pain complaints greater than would be expected from objective clinical findings? ___

   1 = No greater   4 = Marked
   2 = Slight   5 = Extreme
   3 = Moderate   6 = IE

7. In your opinion, will the patient require more, less, or the same level of treatment in the future? a. In the next year: ___ b. Indefinitely: ___

   1 = Less   2 = Same   3 = More

For question 8, please refer to the following definitions:

Sedentary work Jobs such as office worker or clerical position in which the individual spends most of the day sitting but not necessarily sitting continuously for several hours at one time. Workers may be required to stand or walk for brief periods. Lifting requirements are minimal, although the worker may be required occasionally to carry papers, instruments, or books of negligible weight.

Light work Jobs such as retail sales or food service positions in which the worker spends a large amount of time standing or standing/walking. It may also include jobs in which the worker sits most of the time but is required to perform repetitive pushing and pulling of arm or leg controls. Lifting requirements are minimal (maximum 20 pounds), although a worker may be required to frequently lift and carry objects (up to 10 pounds), as in the case of a person who arranges records in filing cabinets or works behind the counter of a variety store wrapping and bagging articles for customers.

Medium work Jobs such as gardener and most custodial positions, in which the worker is required to frequently lift and/or carry items (up to 25 pounds) and occasionally items up to 50 pounds. Lifting and carrying may be performed from a variety of positions, such as squatting or kneeling to change an automobile tire or stooping to assist in lifting persons, pushing litters, and making beds. Jobs in this category also frequently require the worker to stand or stand/walk for extended periods.

Heavy work Jobs such as laborer or warehouse worker, in which workers may be required occasionally to lift and/or carry heavy objects (up to 100 pounds) and frequently carry objects weighing up to 50 pounds. Examples include a worker who pushes a hand truck up and down warehouse aisles while stooping and lifting items with an average weight of 65 pounds and placing them on the hand truck. Jobs in this category also frequently require the worker to standard or stand/walk almost constantly.

8. In your estimation, can this patient work full-time now? ___

    1 = No
    2 = Yes, sedentary work (e.g., stationary job, officer worker)
    3 = Yes, light work (e.g., sales, food service)
    4 = Yes, moderate work (e.g., gardener, custodian)
    5 = Yes, heavy work (e.g., laborer)

    8a. If the answer to question 8 is **No**, in your opinion, will the patient be able to work full-time within the next 6 months? ___

    1 = No
    2 = Yes, sedentary work (e.g., stationary job, officer worker)
    3 = Yes, light work (e.g., sales, food service)
    4 = Yes, moderate work (e.g., gardener, custodian)
    5 = Yes, heavy work (e.g., laborer)

_____   _____
Signature of Physician   Date

General comments and recommendations:

_____
_____
_____
_____

Is there a medical reason why a functional capacity evaluation (FCE) should **not** be performed with this patient? ___ Yes ___ No

Reason:_____

_____

Ending time: _____ A.M./P.M.

4 | Integrated Pain Report

PAIN ASSESSMENT INSTRUMENT

Patient's Name: _____

                                Last   First   Middle Initial

Social Security Number: _ _ _-_ _-_ _ _ _   Today's Date: _ _/_ _/_ _

Instructions

This integrated report format will help you view the patient's pain from multiple perspectives—the patient's, the treating physician's, and the consulting physician's. Insert in the appropriate cell the response given for each of the items. If the cell is shaded, there is no response for that item on the instrument in question.

CP Treating physician form from the Pain Assessment Instrument completed by a second physician

FCE Functional capacity evaluation

PI Patient instrument from the Pain Assessment Instrument

TP Treating physician form from the Pain Assessment Instrument

Description of Variable	PI	TP	CP
Rating of Pain Dimensions			
Frequency of pain (past 6 months)			
Length of pain-free periods (past 6 months)		▓	▓
How long pain lasts (past 6 months)		▓	▓
Unpleasantness during usual pain intensity (past week)		▓	▓
Unpleasantness during highest pain intensity (past week)		▓	▓
Usual intensity of pain			
How often pain awakened you (past 6 months)			
Degree to which patient has talked about pain			
Degree to which patient displays nervousness due to pain	▓		
Medical Information			
Level of joint deformity	▓		
Level of gait abnormalities	▓		

Description of Variable	PI	TP	CP
Amount of support a CT scan gives to complaints	▓		
Amount of support radiographs give to complaints	▓		
Amount of support electrodiagnosis gives to complaints	▓		
Mental Health Status			
How often you felt hopeless (past week)		▓	▓
How often you felt you'd never work again (past week)		▓	▓
How often you felt you'd never do things you enjoyed again		▓	▓
How often you feel depressed (past 6 months)		▓	▓
How severely you felt anxious (past 6 months)		▓	▓
How do you feel about yourself?		▓	▓
How is your appetite now?		▓	▓
Degree to which patient has exhibited mood alterations	▓		
Social Support Networks			
How often significant other becomes irritated because of your pain		▓	▓
How often significant other becomes frustrated because of your pain		▓	▓
Level of difficulty in relationship with spouse or significant other due to pain			
Functional Limitations, Activities of Daily Living			
How much climbing stairs causes pain		▓	
How much bending/stooping/kneeling cause pain		▓	
How much talking/listening cause pain		▓	
How pushing/pulling affect you while in pain		▓	
How climbing stairs affects you while in pain		▓	
How handling/feeling affect you while in pain		▓	
How talking/listening affect you while in pain		▓	
How often pain limited your concentration		▓	
How often pain limited your toleration of minor irritations		▓	
How often you feel frustrated (past 6 months)		▓	▓
How often you attended recreational activities (before pain)		▓	▓
How well can you make decisions now?		▓	▓
Level of difficulty in heavy household tasks due to pain			
Level of difficulty in moving about the house due to pain			
Level of difficulty in traveling independently about town			
Level of difficulty in interpersonal relationships due to pain	▓		
Level of difficulty in remembering instructions due to pain			

Description of Variable	PI	TP	CP
Functional Abilities			
Hours the patient can stand			
Hours the patient can walk			
Hours the patient can push			
Hours the patient can pull			
Hours the patient can stand/walk			
Hours the patient can work overhead			
Hours the patient can sit			
Hours the patient can do simple grasping			
Hours the patient can do fine hand manipulations			
Maximum weight patient can lift floor to counter occasionally			
Maximum weight patient can lift floor to counter repetitively			
Maximum weight patient can lift counter to counter occasionally			
Maximum weight patient can lift counter to counter repetitively			
Maximum weight patient can lift counter to overhead occasionally			
Maximum weight patient can lift counter to overhead repetitively			
Minutes patient can stand without a break			
Minutes patient can sit without a break			
Employment or Rehabilitation Potential			
Level of effort patient will expend for FCE			
When maximum medical improvement can be expected			
Pain complaints greater than from objective clinical findings			
Level of treatment required in the next year			
Level of treatment required in the future (indefinitely)			
Did pain behaviors appear exaggerated?			

Index

Page numbers followed by "f" denote figures; those followed by "t" denote tables.

CHRONIC PAIN EVALUATION: A Valid, Standardized Assessment Instrument discusses how the Pain Assessment Instruments (PAIs) were developed and tested and provides clinical guidelines for their use in an office or administrative setting.

We invite you to help us develop plans for the second phase of this project, which falls into two parts: a national database and the development of software that predicts the likelihood of return to work.

Please circle your responses below and return the completed survey to:

PAI Survey/Medical Division
Butterworth–Heinemann
225 Wildwood Avenue
Woburn, MA 01801-2041
Fax: 781-904-2640
E-mail: PAIsurvey@bhusa.com

Please *rate* the importance of the following:

1. Ability to compare data collected on your patients to other patients in the United States? _____
   a. Not important   b. Important   c. Very important

2. Ability to use the PAI as a measure of treatment effectiveness? _____
   a. Not important   b. Important   c. Very important

3. Ability to enter data directly into a computer? _____
   a. Not important   b. Important   c. Very important

4. Improvement in user friendliness of current form of PAI? _____
   a. Not important   b. Important   c. Very important

5. Ability to predict likelihood of return to work using a user-friendly software program? _____
   a. Not important   b. Important   c. Very important

6. Ability to predict likelihood of return to work by submitting your data to a national site for calculation? _____
   a. Not important   b. Important   c. Very important

7. The accuracy of prediction of return to work? _____
   a. Not important   b. Important   c. Very important

Please tell us about yourself and your practice:

8. Do you have access to the Internet in your office? _____
   a. Yes   b. No

9. Do you use the Internet for clinical use? _____
   a. Yes   b. No

10. Would you prefer to submit data electronically via: _____
    a. Computer disk   b. Website   c. Paper copies of the completed PAI

11. If a system of predicting return to work is made available, for how many patients a year would you use it? _____
    a. <50   b. 50–100   c. 100–300   d. 300–500   e. 500–800   f. 800–1000   g. >1000

12. Are you a (circle as many as applicable):
    a. Health care provider   b. Physician   c. Other: _____

13. Do you work at a (circle as many as applicable):
    a. Pain clinic   b. Rehabilitation hospital/company   c. University   d. Health insurance company
    e. Worker's compensation agency   f. Governmental agency   g. Pharmaceutical company
    h. Other: _____

14. Suggestions for improving user-friendliness of current PAI:

_____

_____

_____

_____

15. Suggestions for elements the national database should feature:

_____

_____

_____

_____

16. Other suggestions and comments:

_____

_____

_____

_____

If you are willing to be contacted for further information regarding the PAI,
please supply the following information:

Name: _____

Institution: _____

Mailing Address: _____

City, State, Zip Code: _____

Phone Number: _____

Fax Number: _____

E-mail Address: _____

Thank you for your time!